Pediatric Endocrinology

Editor

ROBERT RAPAPORT

ENDOCRINOLOGY AND METABOLISM CLINICS OF NORTH AMERICA

www.endo.theclinics.com

Consulting Editor
DEREK LEROITH

December 2012 • Volume 41 • Number 4

ELSEVIER

1600 John F. Kennedy Boulevard • Suite 1800 • Philadelphia, Pennsylvania 19103-2899

http://www.theclinics.com

ENDOCRINOLOGY AND METABOLISM CLINICS OF NORTH AMERICA Volume 41, Number 4
December 2012 ISSN 0889-8529, ISBN-13: 978-1-4557-4841-9

Editor: Pamela Hetherington

Endocrinology and Metabolism Clinics of North America (ISSN 0889-8529) is published quarterly by Elsevier Inc., 360 Park Avenue South, New York, NY 10010-1710. Months of issue are March, June, September, and December. Periodicals postage paid at New York, NY and additional mailing offices. Subscription prices are USD 313.00 per year for US individuals, USD 536.00 per year for US institutions, USD 158.00 per year for US students and residents, USD 393.00 per year for Canadian individuals, USD 656.00 per year for Canadian institutions, USD 456.00 per year for international individuals, USD 656.00 per year for international institutions, and USD 233.00 per year for international and Canadian and foreign students/residents. To receive student/resident rate, orders must be accompanied by name of affiliated institution, date of term, and the signature of program/residency coordinator on institution letterhead. Orders will be billed at individual rate until proof of status is received. Foreign air speed delivery is included in all *Clinics* subscription prices. All prices are subject to change without notice. **POSTMASTER:** Send address changes to *Endocrinology and Metabolism Clinics of North America*, Elsevier Health Sciences Division, Subscription Customer Service, 3251 Riverport Lane, Maryland Heights, MO 63043. **Customer Service: Telephone: 1-800-654-2452** (U.S. and Canada); **1-314-447-8871** (outside U.S. and Canada). **Fax: 1-314-447-8029. E-mail: journalscustomerservice-usa@elsevier.com** (for print support); **journalsonlinesupport-usa@elsevier.com** (for online support).

Reprints. For copies of 100 or more, of articles in this publication, please contact the Commercial Rights Department, Elsevier Inc., 360 Park Avenue South, New York, NY 10010-1710; phone: (+1) 212-633-3813; fax: (+1) 212-462-1935; e-mail: reprints@elsevier.com.

Endocrinology and Metabolism Clinics of North America is covered in *MEDLINE/PubMed (Index Medicus)*, *EMBASE/Excerpta Medica, Current Contents/Clinical Medicine, Current Contents/Life Sciences, Science Citation Index, ISI/BIOMED, BIOSIS,* and *Chemical Abstracts.*

Printed in the United States of America.

Contributors

CONSULTING EDITOR

DEREK LEROITH, MD, PhD
Division of Endocrinology, Metabolism, and Bone Diseases, Department of Medicine,
Mount Sinai School of Medicine, New York, New York

GUEST EDITOR

ROBERT RAPAPORT, MD
Emma Elizabeth Sullivan Professor of Pediatric Endocrinology and Diabetes; Professor
of Pediatrics and Director, Division of Pediatric Endocrinology and Diabetes, Mount Sinai
School of Medicine, New York, New York

AUTHORS

ELIZABETH CHACKO, MD
Fellow, Division of Pediatric Endocrinology and Diabetes, Mount Sinai School of Medicine,
New York, New York

WASSIM CHEMAITILLY, MD
Assistant Member and Director, Division of Endocrinology, Department of Pediatric
Medicine, St. Jude Children's Research Hospital, Memphis, Tennessee

JANE L. CHIANG, MD
Adjunct Assistant Professor, Division of Endocrinology, Department of Pediatrics,
Stanford University, Stanford, California

GERTRUDE COSTIN, MD
Professor of Pediatric Endocrinology Emerita, Keck Medical School, University of
Southern California, Los Angeles, California; Adjunct Professor of Pediatrics, Division
of Pediatric Endocrinology and Diabetes, Mount Sinai School of Medicine, New York,
New York

EVAN GRABER, DO
Fellow, Division of Pediatric Endocrinology and Diabetes, Mount Sinai School of Medicine,
New York, New York

MICHAEL J. HALLER, MD
Associate Professor, Division of Endocrinology, Department of Pediatrics, University
of Florida, Gainesville, Florida

STEPHEN F. KEMP, MD, PhD
Professor of Pediatrics, Arkansas Children's Hospital, University of Arkansas for Medical
Sciences, Little Rock, Arkansas

LIORA LAZAR, MD
The Jesse Z and Sara Lea Shafer Institute for Endocrinology and Diabetes, National Center for Childhood Diabetes, Schneider Children's Medical Center of Israel, Petach Tikva, Israel; Sackler Faculty of Medicine, Tel Aviv University, Tel Aviv, Israel

TERRI H. LIPMAN, PhD, CRNP
Division of Endocrinology and Diabetes, The Children's Hospital of Philadelphia; Professor of Nursing of Children, Department of Family and Community Health, University of Pennsylvania School of Nursing, Philadelphia, Pennsylvania

KATHERINE LORD, MD
Fellow, Division of Endocrinology and Diabetes, The Children's Hospital of Philadelphia, Philadelphia, Pennsylvania

MOSHE PHILLIP, MD
The Jesse Z and Sara Lea Shafer Institute for Endocrinology and Diabetes, National Center for Childhood Diabetes, Schneider Children's Medical Center of Israel, Petach Tikva, Israel; Sackler Faculty of Medicine, Tel Aviv University, Tel Aviv, Israel

ALBA MORALES POZZO, MD
Associate Professor of Pediatrics, Arkansas Children's Hospital, University of Arkansas for Medical Sciences, Little Rock, Arkansas

ROBERT RAPAPORT, MD
Emma Elizabeth Sullivan Professor of Pediatric Endocrinology and Diabetes; Professor of Pediatrics and Director, Division of Pediatric Endocrinology and Diabetes, Mount Sinai School of Medicine, New York, New York

MOLLY O. REGELMANN, MD
Attending, Division of Pediatric Endocrinology and Diabetes, Mount Sinai School of Medicine, New York, New York

LESLIE L. ROBISON, PhD
Chair, Department of Epidemiology and Cancer Control, St. Jude Children's Research Hospital, Memphis, Tennessee

DESMOND A. SCHATZ, MD
Professor and Associate Chair, Division of Endocrinology, Department of Pediatrics, University of Florida, Gainesville, Florida

DIANA E. STANESCU, MD
Fellow, Division of Endocrinology and Diabetes, The Children's Hospital of Philadelphia, Philadelphia, Pennsylvania

CONSTANTINE A. STRATAKIS, MD, D (Med) Sci
Scientific Director and Director, Pediatric Endocrinology Training Program; Section on Endocrinology and Genetics, Program in Developmental Endocrinology and Genetics, *Eunice Kennedy Shriver* National Institute of Child Health and Human Development, National Institutes of Health, Bethesda, Maryland

ALFRED TENORE, MD
Professor of Pediatrics, Division of Pediatric Endocrinology, Department of Pediatrics, DSMSC, University of Udine, Udine, Italy; President, European Academy of Paediatrics, Paediatric Section of UEMS, Brussels, Belgium

ANDREW TENORE, MD
Division of Pediatric Endocrinology, Department of Pediatrics, DSMSC, University of Udine, Udine, Italy

ELIZABETH WALLACH, MD
Attending, Division of Pediatric Endocrinology and Diabetes, Mount Sinai School of Medicine, New York, New York

Contents

Diana E. Stanescu, Katherine Lord, and Terri H. Lipman

Type 1 diabetes is one of the most common chronic diseases of childhood and adolescence. Multiple registries have assessed its epidemiology and have noted a steady increase in incidence of the disease. This article addresses the epidemiology of type 1 diabetes in children aged 0 to 19 years, by reviewing the available, current data from both US and international registries. The prevalence and incidence data by race, ethnicity, age of onset, sex, season of onset, and temporal trends of the disease are presented. Multiple risk factors have been implicated for the increasing incidence in type 1 diabetes, and these genetic and environmental risk factors are discussed.

Jane L. Chiang, Michael J. Haller, and Desmond A. Schatz

Remarkable progress has been made in strategies to arrest pancreatic β-cell destruction in type 1 diabetes. Although knowledge of the disease has increased, a safe therapeutic intervention to reverse or prevent it remains elusive. The interaction of genes, immune system, and environment result in a complex disease process that has delayed hopes for a cure. Several well-designed prevention and intervention studies have aspired to test potentially efficacious and safe therapies. This article updates the principles used to design prevention and intervention trials, reviews clinical trials, addresses controversial issues, and provides a framework for future efforts to interdict this condition.

Elizabeth Chacko, Evan Graber, Molly O. Regelmann, Elizabeth Wallach, Gertrude Costin, and Robert Rapaport

Turner syndrome (TS) and Noonan syndrome (NS) have short stature as a constant feature; however, both conditions can present clinicians with a challenging array of genetic, cardiovascular, developmental, and psychosocial issues. In recent years, important advances have been achieved in each of these areas. This article reviews these two syndromes and provides updates on recent developments in diagnostic evaluation, growth and development, psychological issues, and treatment options for patients with TS and NS.

treatment of endogenous Cushing syndrome. It also discusses the clinical and molecular genetics of inherited forms of this syndrome. Cushing syndrome needs to be diagnosed and treated properly when first recognized; improper treatment can turn this otherwise completely curable disorder into a chronic ailment. Barriers to optimal care of a pediatric patient with Cushing syndrome are discussed.

Bone age (BA) indicates more clearly than chronologic age how far an individual has progressed toward full maturity, and predicts the potential for further growth. Single or serial skeletal age estimations help to confirm the diagnosis of normal puberty and normal pubertal variants such as constitutional delay of growth and puberty, premature therlache, and precocious adrenarche. BA can aid in the clinical workup of children whose sexual maturation is early or delayed. Although BA is considered a qualitative rather than quantitative measure, it serves to round out the clinical picture, providing information without which diagnosis could not be achieved.

ENDOCRINOLOGY AND METABOLISM CLINICS OF NORTH AMERICA

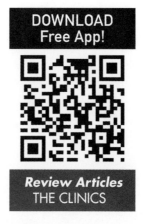

Foreword

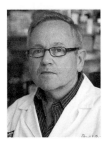

Derek LeRoith, MD, PhD
Consulting Editor

As the readers are well aware, our understanding of endocrine disorders is constantly in flux as new research, both basic and clinical, is presented. Thus it is always timely to review and update the readers on various topics, in this case, Pediatric Endocrine Disorders.

The issue begins with an article by Drs Stanescu, Lord, and Lipman, who discuss the epidemiology of type 1 diabetes. Most registries show that the prevalence of type 1 diabetes ranges from ∼1.5 to 2.0 cases per 1000 individuals, the highest being in Caucasians and Southeast Asians, and between racial and ethnic groups there are large variations. The incidence is apparently highest around puberty, perhaps due to hormonal influences. Overall there is a distinct increase incidence of type 1 diabetes over the past decade or two, and this has also shown up in the very young age group. The etiology remains an enigma with a clear genetic component and questionable environmental factors being involved. These include viral infections and toxins. The influence of milk, diet, vitamin D status, and obesity remains unclear.

Of particular interest over the past decade have been the multicenter, international interventional studies that have been conducted to "prevent" or intervene in early stages of type 1 diabetes. As Drs Chiang, Haller, and Schatz discuss, while the studies are well planned and executed, the success in overcoming the immunological aspect of the disease remains an issue. They summarize trials like the DPT1, DIPP, and numerous others, run by the Trialnet collaborative study groups. While the success rate has been modest, they conclude that the depth of understanding of the autoimmune process, the international collaborative effect, should bring us closer to finding the "cure," which must involve dealing with the autoimmunity.

Drs Pozo and Kemp remind us in their article that GH has been available since the 1950s for the treatment of GH deficiency. While the FDA has approved its use in GH deficiency, ISS, Turners, and other non-GH-deficiency states, there are others that have been studied where GH maybe beneficial. In their article they discuss the use of GH in cystic fibrosis, and chronic inflammatory disorders, such as juvenile idiopathic arthritis and Crohns. Its value in burn cases, small bowel syndrome, thalassemia,

Endocrinol Metab Clin N Am 41 (2012) xi–xiii
http://dx.doi.org/10.1016/j.ecl.2012.08.005
0889-8529/12/$ – see front matter © 2012 Published by Elsevier Inc.

hyphosphatemic rickets, and chronic kidney disease has also been discussed. However, the authors conclude that, despite the positive effects and relative safety profile, more studies are required to establish the appropriate usage of GH therapy in these conditions.

Drs Chacko, Regelmann, Graben, Costin, and Rapaport described the growth retardation associated with Turner and Noonan syndrome. While each syndrome has different genetic, developmental, and cardiac aspects, they both respond to the FDA-approved GH therapy. Interestingly, while adult height is positively affected by GH in Turner syndrome, in the case of Noonan syndrome this remains to be determined. Nevertheless, growth-retarded children should be screened for these syndromes since GH therapy maybe indicated.

Drs Tenore and Tenore discuss a very perplexing disorder, namely attention-deficient hyperactivity disorder (ADHD) and whether the disorder is associated with growth effects and/or whether the commonly used medication to treat ADHD causes arrested growth, even temporarily. The article delves quite deeply in both the disorder and the medications that are used and, in their opinion, the studies are so varied that it is hard to conclude how much growth retardation occurs, whether secondary to the ADHD or the medications.

Following cranial radiotherapy for cancer in childhood, GH deficiency is a common phenomenon and GH replacement therapy is an important therapeutic option. On the other hand, since GH and particularly IGF-1 have mitogenic activities, there is a significant concern about potential side effects, particularly cancer growth, as discussed by Drs Chemaitilly and Robison. However, its use in childhood cancer survivors has not been proven to cause recurrence or worsen survival. When GH is used in children that have received radiation, there is apparently an increased incidence of meningiomas; therefore, it is prudent to follow those postradiation individuals on GH replacement more closely.

Down syndrome is a relatively common disorder in the United States and worldwide and is often associated with thyroid dysfunction. As discussed in the article by Graber, Costin, and Rapaport, congenital hypothyroidism, autoimmune hypothyroidism, and Graves disease occur not uncommonly in these children. In addition, mild hypothyroidism may present with elevated TSH levels and normal thyroid function. Most importantly, patients with Down syndrome should be screened with repeated TSH measurements of TSH and treated appropriately, since the classic signs and symptoms of thyroid disorders should not be be used as clinical indications of thyroid disorders since they are commonly seen in Down syndrome in the absence of thyroid disease.

In Dr Stratakis' article we learn that while Cushings syndrome is common secondary to exogenous glucocorticoid usage, there are genetic forms of the disorder. Furthermore, careful attention should be paid to making the correct diagnosis so as not to allow the condition to become a chronic ailment. This can be achieved by a better understanding of the hypothalamic-pituitary-adrenal axis and by using the appropriate tests. Surgery and specific medications have been well tested and, when used correctly by experienced physicians, offer outstanding results. Bone maturation is the natural phenomenon occurring during puberty, whereby the fusion of the growth plate is the final process in longitudinal bone growth. During the pubertal growth spurt there is a more rapid maturation of bone age, as described in the article by Drs Lazar and Phillip. Furthermore, it is important to realize that in normal puberty there is often a discordance between bone age and timing of pubertal stages and similarly in boys with precocious puberty. Another measure that is critical is the adult height prediction in evaluating the need for therapy in cases of either precocious or delayed puberty.

Dr Rapaport has collected a number of important articles for this issue that we are sure pediatricians and pediatric endocrinologists will find very useful in their practice and we are grateful to the authors for their outstanding contributions.

Derek LeRoith, MD, PhD
Division of Endocrinology, Metabolism, and Bone Diseases
Department of Medicine
Mount Sinai School of Medicine
One Gustave L. Levy Place
Box 1055, Altran 4-36
New York, NY 10029, USA

E-mail address:
derek.leroith@mssm.edu

Preface

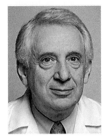

Robert Rapaport, MD
Guest Editor

Knowledge in the field of medicine is expanding at a rapid rate. Pediatric Endocrinology is no exception. New developments in hormonal disorders affecting children are accruing at an increasingly faster pace. Therefore having another addition of the *Endocrinology and Metabolism Clinics of North America* dedicated to issues in pediatric endocrinology is most appropriate at this time.

While in the previous issues we discussed the growing epidemic of obesity and related type 2 diabetes, it is important to remember that still the most common form of diabetes affecting children is type 1 diabetes. Therefore contributions dedicated to the changing epidemiology of type 1 diabetes as well as an update on means of prevention of type 1 diabetes in youth are featured at the outset.

Growth is the single most common cause for referral to a pediatric endocrinologist. While in previous issues we have discussed an overview of growth and growth hormone treatment and some of the common conditions for which growth hormone is currently prescribed, in this issue of the *Endocrinology and Metabolism Clinics of North America* we tackle some of the nontraditional conditions for which growth hormone therapy may or may not be helpful and conditions for which, although some reports have documented use, are not FDA approved. In addition, less common conditions for which growth hormone is currently FDA approved, such as Turner and Noonan syndrome, are reviewed with an emphasis on new management concepts.

An ever-increasing segment of the pediatric population is diagnosed with attention deficit and hyperactivity disorder. Whether this condition is associated with growth issues or whether the medications used for its treatment have an impact on children's growth is very controversial. An erudite review of the topic will help the reader frame, if not answers, at least some of the questions surrounding this condition.

First and foremost in pediatric care is the caution to do no harm to children. For that reason an update on the safety of growth hormone therapy, especially in children who have had previous malignancy, is included.

Down syndrome is a relatively common disorder identified in the pediatric population. Frequently these children are evaluated for possible thyroid dysfunction; therefore, that subject will be reviewed in this issue as well.

Endocrinol Metab Clin N Am 41 (2012) xv–xvi
http://dx.doi.org/10.1016/j.ecl.2012.08.006
0889-8529/12/$ – see front matter © 2012 Elsevier Inc. All rights reserved.

With the increasing rate of obesity, one of the conditions that needs to be excluded in children with obesity is Cushing syndrome. While it is not a very common condition in pediatrics, it is an extremely important one to be both identified as well as treated properly. Therefore a state-of-the-art update article on the diagnosis and management of Cushing syndrome is included.

Utilized and perhaps overutilized in the evaluation and management of children with growth and pubertal disorders are bone age assessments. A detailed review of the proper perspective of bone age evaluations is provided in a separate article.

I would like to thank the editor of the *Endocrinology and Metabolism Clinics of North America*, Dr Leroith, as well as the publishers for allowing and promoting an ongoing report on selected advances in the field of Pediatric Endocrinology. Last and most importantly, I would like to express my sincere appreciation to all the expert contributors whose hard work made the production of this volume possible.

Robert Rapaport, MD
Division of Pediatric Endocrinology and Diabetes
Mount Sinai School of Medicine
One Gustave L. Levy Place, Box 1616
New York, NY 10029, USA

E-mail address:
robert.rapaport@mountsinai.org

Erratum

Please note that the affiliation for Dr Sol Epstein in the September 2012 issue of Endocrinology and Metabolism Clinics is incorrect. His affiliation should read:

Sol Epstein, MD, FRCP, FACP
Professor of Medicine and Geriatrics
Mt. Sinai School of Medicine
New York, NY

Adjunct Professor of Medicine
University of Pennsylvania Medical School
Philadelphia, PA

Endocrinol Metab Clin N Am 41 (2012) xvii
http://dx.doi.org/10.1016/j.ecl.2012.10.001
0889-8529/12/$ – see front matter © 2012 Elsevier Inc. All rights reserved.

The Epidemiology of Type 1 Diabetes in Children

Diana E. Stanescu, MD[a], Katherine Lord, MD[a],
Terri H. Lipman, PhD, CRNP[a,b,*]

KEYWORDS

- Type 1 diabetes • Children • Incidence • Prevalence • Risk factors

KEY POINTS

- The incidence of type 1 diabetes is increasing.
- The risk factors for the development of type 1 diabetes are still controversial.
- A national system of surveillance is necessary to determine the true epidemiology of type 1 diabetes.

INTRODUCTION

Diabetes is a wonderful affection, not very frequent among men, being a melting down of the flesh and limbs into urine...
— *Aretaeus the Cappadocian, second century AD*

Diabetes is an ancient disease yet much about the disorder is still unknown. The key to the understanding of diabetes is a thorough knowledge of the extent of its existence. This article reviews the epidemiology of type 1 diabetes mellitus in children and adolescents worldwide. Type 1 diabetes is the third most prevalent chronic disease of childhood in the United States; only asthma and obesity are more common.[1] The risk of devastating complications remains high. Diabetes is the leading cause of nephropathy, retinopathy, neuropathy, and coronary and peripheral vascular disease and represents an enormous public health burden. The annual cost of type 1 diabetes in the United States is $14.4 billion.[2] The incidence of type 1 diabetes in children is increasing, and knowledge of the temporal trends and the geographic,

Disclosures: The authors have nothing to disclose.
Funding sources: None.
[a] Division of Endocrinology and Diabetes, The Children's Hospital of Philadelphia, 34th and Civic Center Blvd, Philadelphia, PA 19104, USA; [b] Department of Family and Community Health, University of Pennsylvania School of Nursing, 418 Curie Boulevard, Philadelphia, PA 19104, USA
* Corresponding author. Department of Family and Community Health, University of Pennsylvania School of Nursing, 418 Curie Boulevard, Philadelphia, PA 19104.
E-mail address: lipman@nursing.upenn.edu

Endocrinol Metab Clin N Am 41 (2012) 679–694
http://dx.doi.org/10.1016/j.ecl.2012.08.001
0889-8529/12/$ – see front matter © 2012 Elsevier Inc. All rights reserved.

endo.theclinics.com

demographic, and biologic differences in incidence is necessary in elucidating the multifactorial cause of the disease. Despite the severity and impact of type 1 diabetes, it has only been since the end of the 20th century that the epidemiology of type 1 diabetes has been intensively investigated through a joint international effort to map the global patterns of this disease.

Although others have reviewed the epidemiology of type 1 diabetes across the lifespan,[3] this article is limited to type 1 diabetes in youth. An overview and the history of collaborative registries will be presented. The prevalence of type 1 diabetes is described. The overall incidence rates of type 1 diabetes in the United States, and globally, are discussed. In addition, data related to differences in incidence by age, race, and ethnicity and season of onset, as well as the temporal trends of the disease, are presented. The article will conclude with an overview of the genetic and environmental risk factors of type 1 diabetes.

REGISTRIES OF TYPE 1 DIABETES IN CHILDREN

Population-based registries are the most comprehensive methods to obtain complete data on disease incidence and to monitor temporal trends. It has been recognized that rigorous epidemiologic methods were needed to obtain standardized data on the incidence of diabetes. The early work on registries of type 1 diabetes was developed through the Diabetes Epidemiology Research International group.[4] This group identified broad international variation and the suggestion of temporal variation in incidence. In the early 1990s, the World Health Organization (WHO) began its Multinational Project for Childhood Diabetes (DIAMOND Study [Diabetes Mondiale]). The essence of this project was the establishment of population-based registries with a formal assessment of ascertainment. It was composed of a consortium of 150 registries in 70 countries, using the same methodology for the purpose of obtaining standardized data for comparison.[5] These registries monitored the global incidence of type 1 diabetes, evaluated risk factors for geographic and temporal variation, assessed mortality, and evaluated socioeconomic factors related to type 1 diabetes.[6] The DIAMOND project reported a greater than 350-fold difference in the incidence of diabetes in children worldwide.[7]

In the 1990s, 14 registries of type 1 diabetes in children in the United States were actively collecting data using the WHO criteria. Longstanding pediatric diabetes registries in the United States include those from Allegheny County, PA, USA,[8] and Chicago, IL, USA.[9] More recently, the SEARCH for Diabetes in Youth Study was developed, collecting data from 10 study locations for children with diabetes, beginning in 2002, using different methodology than the registries in the DIAMOND study.[10] The Philadelphia Pediatric Diabetes Registry is the only remaining registry in the country continuously collecting and publishing incidence data on black, white, and Hispanic children with type 1 diabetes since 1985.[11]

The Europe and Diabetes Study (EURODIAB), which includes 44 European centers, has been collecting data since the 1980s, which have demonstrated a widespread, marked increase in type 1 diabetes during the course of the study.[12] Establishment of population-based registries of type 1 around the world is necessary to monitor the global pattern of the disease and to provide a basis for standardized studies of risk factors.

PREVALENCE

Few studies have examined the prevalence of type 1 diabetes in youth because of inherent difficulties in case assessment and study period variability. Most prevalence estimates are calculated based on cumulative incidence rates. Based on this methodology, it was estimated that in 2011, 490,000 children younger than 15 years had type 1 diabetes worldwide.[13] The global distribution of type 1 diabetes varies significantly by region. Europe is estimated to have the largest number of prevalent type 1 diabetes cases, followed closely by Southeast Asia, including India. The West Pacific region, including China, has the lowest number of prevalent type 1 diabetes cases.[13]

The most extensive examination of type 1 diabetes prevalence in youth comes from the SEARCH for Diabetes in Youth study.[14] This study of the US population estimated the prevalence of type 1 diabetes at 1.54 cases/1000 youth. Prevalence was highest among non-Hispanic whites aged 10 to 19 years, with 2.88 cases/1000 youth, followed by blacks aged 10 to 19 years, with 2.07 cases/1000 youth. Overall, no gender differences in the prevalence of type 1 diabetes were found. However, higher rates in girls were noted in 3 racial/ethnic groups: black, Asian/Pacific Islander, and American Indian. A population-based survey of the Philadelphia region found a similar overall type 1 diabetes prevalence of 1.58/1000 youth. By racial group, the prevalence of type 1 diabetes was 2.69/1000 non-Hispanic white youth, 1.02/1000 African American youth, and 1.70/1000 Hispanic youth.[15] Other regions that have published data on type 1 diabetes prevalence include Sardinia (4.64/1000), Manitoba, Canada (1.2/1000), Saudi Arabia (1.1/1000), and Istanbul, Turkey (0.67/1000).[16–19]

Incidence in the United States

The first US registry of pediatric type 1 diabetes–the Allegheny County registry–began collecting data in 1965 and reported an overall age-standardized annual incidence rate of 16.7/100,000 in the last published cohort of 1990–1994.[8] The Chicago Childhood Diabetes Registry analyzed hospital data from a 10-year period, between 1994 and 2003, and estimated an overall annual incidence rate of type 1 diabetes of 10.8/100,000 boys and 11.5/100,000 girls aged 0 to 17 years.[9] In its more recent analysis of cases diagnosed between 2000 and 2004, the Philadelphia registry reports an overall age-adjusted annual incidence of 16/100,000 children aged 0 to 14 years.[11]

The recent SEARCH study evaluated youth younger than 20 years who were newly diagnosed with diabetes between 2002 and 2005, from 10 sites in 4 US geographic regions. They reported an overall annual incidence of diabetes of 24.3/100,000 between 2002 and 2003; approximately 70% of these cases were classified as type 1 diabetes.[10] A subsequent analysis of new cases diagnosed between 2002 and 2005 estimated an overall annual incidence of type 1 diabetes 19.7/100,000 in children younger than 10 years and of 18.6/100,000 for the 10- to 19-year-olds.[20]

Geographic Variation in the United States

Although there is no estimate of type 1 diabetes incidence for every US state, the location of different registries can provide useful information on geographic variation. Two registries, the Philadelphia and Allegheny county registries, located in the same state, recorded annual incidence rates for the 1990–1994 interval: 13.1/100,000 (confidence interval, 11.4–14.9) for children aged 0 to 14 years and 16.7/100,000 (confidence interval, 14.7–18.8) for children aged 0 to 19 years, respectively.[8,11]

The SEARCH study analyzed the incidence rate in 4 other states. The highest crude incidence rate among all races was recorded in 10- to 14-year- old children in Colorado (33/100,000 per year) and Ohio (36/100,000 per year), followed by Washington and South Carolina (22.3/100,000 per year).[21] The Philadelphia registry showed a lower incidence rate of 19.9/100,000 per year in this age group and time period. In the 15- to 19-year-old group, Washington and Ohio had the highest incidence (15/100,000), followed by Colorado and South Carolina with the lowest rate (6.7/100,000).[21]

Overall, the distribution of incident type 1 diabetes cases in the United States does not show a similar geographic distribution as that in Europe, with a higher incidence in the northern regions and a lower one in the south. This is possibly because of the heterogeneous racial background of US population compared with the more geographically stable European populations. However, even when comparing apparently racially homogeneous populations, diagnosed in the same period of time and of the same age, variations in incidence rates still persist, suggesting the involvement of other factors (**Table 1**).

International Incidence and Trends

The analysis of type 1 diabetes incidence worldwide is an extremely arduous task. The geographic variations are caused by the multitude of factors that contribute to the pathogenesis of type 1 diabetes and the difficulties in diagnosing and reporting this disease in different regions and countries.

The first global diabetes incidence study, the WHO DIAMOND Project, collected data between 1990 and 1999 and reported incidence data for children younger than 14 years of age from 112 centers in 57 countries. A total of 43,013 children of a study population of 84 million were diagnosed with type 1 diabetes during this time. The overall incidence varied more than 350-fold among countries in the same region and between regions–from 0.1/100,000 per year in China and Venezuela to 37.8/100,000 per year in Sardinia to 40.9/100,000 per year in Finland.[7] The more recent EURODIAB Study collected data from 17 countries in children younger than 15 years between 1989 and 2003. The highest incidence was reported in Finland at 52.6% (per 100,000) and lowest in Lithuania (10.3/100,000).[12]

It is estimated that approximately 78,000 children worldwide develop type 1 diabetes annually. Europe and Southeast Asia are the regions with the highest estimated number of new type 1 diabetes cases in children 0 to 14 years of age, representing approximately 18,000 cases per year for each. Most of the new cases diagnosed in Southeast Asia are from India, with an overall annual estimated incidence rate of 4.2/100,000. The highest incidence is estimated in Finland, followed by Sweden, Sardinia, Saudi Arabia, Norway, and the United Kingdom (**Fig. 1**).[13,22]

Incidence of Type 1 Diabetes by Age at Onset

The age distribution of incidence rates for type 1 diabetes suggests that the age of onset increases during childhood and then steadily decreases toward adulthood (**Table 2**).[7,10,12] It is generally accepted that hormonal changes at puberty are responsible for the highest incidence in 10- to 14-year-old children compared with other age

Table 1
Geographic variation in incidence rate in 10- to 14-year-old children in 5 US states

	Incidence Rate				
	South Carolina[21]	Colorado[21]	Ohio[21]	Washington[21]	Philadelphia, PA[11]
Non-Hispanic white	27.6	39.3	40.3	32.4	22.6
African American	14.7	–	–	16.2	16.8
Hispanic	–	19.9	–	–	17.8

The rates are reported in new cases per 100,000 per year. The SEARCH study[21] represents new cases diagnosed between 2002 and 2003. The Philadelphia registry data[11] represent newly diagnosed cases between 2000 and 2004.

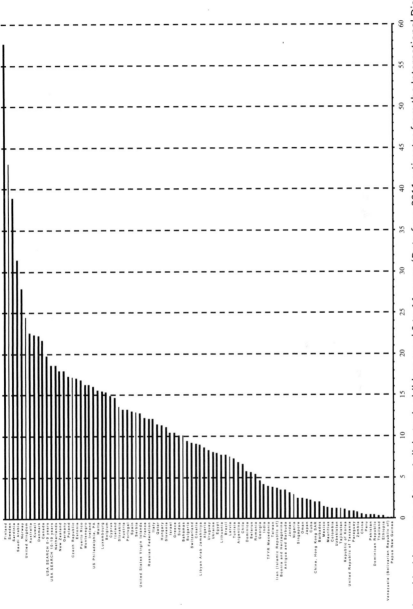

Fig. 1. International incidence rate of type 1 diabetes in children aged 0 to 14 years. (*Data from* 2011 estimates from the International Diabetes Federation,[13] Sardinia,[22] and the SEARCH and Philadelphia registries for US data[7,11]).

Table 2
Incidence rates by age group in 8 registries

Registry	Study Period	Age Group, y			
		0–4	5–9	10–14	15–19
Philadelphia, PA[29,30,32]	1985–1990	21%	37%	41%	–
	1990–1994	7.4 (21%)	13.6 (33%)	18.9 (46%)	–
	1995–1999	7.4 (18%)	16.7 (37%)	20.7 (45%)	–
Allegheny, PA[8]	1990–1994	8.6 (14%)	19.2 (31%)	24.3 (36%)	12.3 (20%)
Chicago, IL[9]	1994–2003	7.6 (20%)	12.7 (33%)	13.8 (32.5%)	10.4 (14%) (15–17 y)
SEARCH[10]	2002–2003	14.3 (18%)	22.1 (28%)	25.9 (36%)	13.1 (17%)
EURODIAB[12]	1989–2003	24%	35%	41%	–

The incidence is reported in new cases per 100,000 per year and in percentage of total number of new cases (in parentheses and italics).

groups. The peak of incidence for girls seems to occur 3 years before the peak of incidence for boys.[23]

Recent cohorts show a trend toward a higher incidence rate overall, with children younger than 10 years having significantly higher rates of developing diabetes. In its last cohort, 2000 to 2004, the Philadelphia registry showed a dramatic increase in incidence in children aged 0 to 4 years compared with the 1990 to 1994 cohort. The rate in black children aged 0 to 4 years was 2.5 higher in the 2000 to 2004 cohort compared with the 1990 to 1994 cohort. Furthermore, the incidence in children aged 5 to 9 years seemed to approach the incidence in children aged 10 to 14 years, suggesting a flattening of the age differences.[11]

A similar trend of increasing incidence in younger age groups was seen in both EURODIAB and DIAMOND studies.[12,13] However, these trends are not uniform among countries. For example, New Zeeland, with a population of mostly European ancestry and a moderate overall incidence rate, reported the highest increase in increase in incidence in children aged 10 to 14 years and the lowest increase among children aged 0 to 4 years.[24]

Incidence of Type 1 Diabetes by Sex

The distribution of incidence rates between male and female children varies greatly by the reporting region or registry, but also by the age, race, and the years the data were collected. Although diabetes, as an autoimmune disease, would be expected to have a higher incidence in girls, there is a slightly higher incidence rate for boys, especially in non-Hispanic white children, in several US registries.[8,9,25]

In the SEARCH data, the incidence of type 1 diabetes was higher in African American girls aged 10 to 14 years and in Hispanic and non-Hispanic white girls aged 5 to 9 years than in boys.[26] The analysis of a large Finnish cohort, diagnosed during a period of 25 years (1980–2005), showed the same overall 1:1 ratio between boys and girls aged 0 to 15 but a significant divergence after the age of 13, when the ratio became 1.7:1.[23]

On a larger scale, EURODIAB analyzed the incidence trends during 15 years and found a more rapid increase in incidence in girls aged 5 to 9 years and slower in girls aged 10 to 14 years compared with boys. Boys aged 10 to 14 years tended to have had a higher risk than same age girls of being newly diagnosed to diabetes in central and eastern European countries, with a more accelerated increase in incidence rates than the rest of Europe.[12]

Racial and Ethnic Differences in the Incidence of Type 1 Diabetes

Incidence in non-Hispanic white youth
In general, non-Hispanic white youth are the racial group with the highest incidence of type 1 diabetes, but there are several important regional and temporal differences among US registries. The Allegheny County registry, reporting data from 1965 to 1989 in 0- to 19-year-old children, calculated an annual incidence rate of 14.1/100,000 in white children, higher than in blacks.[27] In the last cohort that was reported, 1990 to 1994, the annual incidence in whites was 16.5/100,000, slightly lower than the incidence in nonwhites of 17.6/100,000. The Chicago registry (1994–2003) also reported higher incidence rates in 0- to 17-year-old whites compared with other racial groups: 16.2 and 14.3/100,000 in boys and girls, respectively.[9] The most recent cohort of the Philadelphia registry (2000–2004) reported an annual incidence rate in children younger than 14 years of 18.2/100,000, lower than the incidence in Hispanic children in this area.[11] The SEARCH study estimated an overall incidence of 23.6/100,000 for white children aged 0 to 19 years and 27.5/100,000 in those aged 0 to 14 years, and about 30% were overweight or obese and came from families with higher socioeconomic status than newly diagnosed children with type 2 diabetes.[26]

The European incidence rates, for the same age group and racial background, varied between 40.9 in Finland (highest incidence in Europe) and 5.3 in Romania (lowest incidence in Europe) in 1990 to 1999. In some geographic areas, the incidence of type 1 diabetes in white US children is among the highest in the world.

Incidence in black youth
The incidence of type 1 diabetes in black children is generally lower than that in non-Hispanic white children, but seems to vary greatly between registries and to have markedly increased in some areas of the United States This trend is thought to be related to an overall increase in type 1 diabetes incidence, a more diverse cause and pathogenesis of diabetes, changes in environmental factors, or increased rates of obesity in black children and adolescents.[8]

In its first cohort in 1965 to 1976, the Allegheny county registry reported an annual incidence rate of 10.1/100,000 in black boys and 11/100,000/year in black girls aged 0 to 19 years.[28] By the time of the last cohort published, 1990 to 1994, the overall annual incidence rate increased to 17.6/100,000 for nonwhite children, of which 95% were black, surpassing for the first time the incidence in white children. The 15- to 19-year-old nonwhite youth had the highest recorded annual incidence rates: 30.4/100,000 between 1990 and 1994 compared with only 7.6/100,000 between 1980 and 1984, or compared with 11.2/100,000 in white youth of the same age between 1990 and 1994.[8]

The overall incidence in the Philadelphia for black children aged 0 to 14 years was estimated at 12.8/100,000, between 1990 and 1994, with no significant differences between boys and girls. In the same cohort, black children aged 10 to 14 years had a higher risk of developing type 1 diabetes compared with other racial groups.[29] A subsequent analysis of the same population between 1995 and 1999 showed an incidence rate of 15.4/100,000, for the first time surpassing the rate in white children. The same pattern of increased incidence in 10- to 14-year-old children remained (26.9 in black children compared with 11.3/100,000 in white children). The incidence of 14.9/100,000 in children aged 5 to 9 years was the highest rate ever reported to that date.[30] The most recent data analysis of the Philadelphia Registry, between

2000 and 2004, shows an overall annual incidence in black children of 13.6/100,000, lower than the incidence in white or Hispanic children in all age groups under study.

The SEARCH study, in analyzing a much larger cohort of newly diagnosed cases in a greater geographic area between 2002 and 2005, found lower incidence rates of type 1 diabetes in African American children than in white children: 19.3/100,000 for children aged 5 to 9 years, 21.3/100,000 for children aged 10 to 14 years, and 9.5/100,000 for children aged 15 to 19 years. In the SEARCH cohort, African American girls were more commonly diagnosed than boys and they also had higher percentages of overweight and obesity. Overall, 44.7% of African American children with type 1 diabetes were overweight or obese.

The socioeconomic analysis showed that these children lived in households with lower annual income (33% vs ~10% of white children are part of families with <$25,000 annual income).[26]

Incidence in Hispanic American youth

The incidence of type 1 diabetes in Hispanic American youth also varies greatly between reporting registries and studied time periods and depends on the country of origin of different populations. One of the first studies reporting incidence data in Hispanic children analyzed different ethnic groups in San Diego, CA, USA, between 1978 and 1981. The number of new cases in Mexican American children was 8 times lower than in Caucasian children aged 0 to 19 years.[31]

Another recent analysis compared incidence rates in 0- to 17-year-old Colorado youth between 1978 and 1988 (Colorado IDDM Study Registry) and 2002 to 2004 (SEARCH study data). The incidence rate in Hispanic American children was 10.7/100,000 per year for girls and 7.5/100,000 per year for boys in the first cohort. The incidence rates increased by 1.6% per year between the 2 cohorts, compared with 2.7% increase in non-Hispanic white youth. Overall, children aged 10 to 14 years had higher incidence rates compared with other age groups, similar to age patterns seen in nonwhite Hispanic children.[25]

The Philadelphia Registry has consistently reported during the past 20 years the highest incidence rates of type 1 diabetes in Hispanic children, compared with other racial groups in this region. Between 1985 and 1999, the incidence of type 1 diabetes in Hispanic children has remained relatively stable: 15.16 (1985–1989), 15.5 (1990–1994), and 15.6 (1995–1999).[29,30,32] More recently, the incidence rate increased to 17.8/100,000 per year between 2000 and 2004, still higher than the incidence rates in the other racial subgroups.[11] The reason for the higher incidence rates in Hispanic children in Philadelphia is that the vast majority of the Hispanic children living in this area are of Puerto Rican descent. The incidence rates in Puerto Rico are also the highest in the South and Central American region. Between 1985 and 1994, the incidence rate was 18.0/100,000 per year, with slight female predominance and no difference between various areas of the island.[33] The DIAMOND project reported an incidence rate of 16.8/100,000 per year between 1990 and 1999, similar to those in the Philadelphia region but much higher than other Hispanic countries in the region: 1.5 in Mexico or 0.1 in Venezuela[7] The Puerto Rican population has a diverse genetic background: 50% to 55% for southern European, 29% to 30% for western African, and 15% to 20% for Amerindian, northern European, or Asian; this genetic background is possibly responsible for this higher incidence rates.[33]

The SEARCH study reported an incidence in Hispanic youths aged 0 to 14 years of 15.0/100,000 per year in girls and 16.2/100,000 per year in boys, between 2002 and 2005. Most of these children were of Mexican or Mexican American descent (55%), whereas other Central and South American counties of origin were less well represented. And 44% of them were overweight and obese.[34] When compared with DIAMOND data, these incidence rates were much higher than those reported in Mexico and the South and Central American region overall (5.8/100,000).[7]

In regions with a more homogeneous Hispanic population, the type 1 diabetes incidence rates tend to be similar to the incidence in their country of origin. However, in regions with a more heterogeneous population, the incidence rates are much higher than would be predicted just based on their country of origin. More specifically, it seems that Puerto Rican youth are the only Hispanic subgroup whose migration to mainland United States does not result in higher incidence rates. These findings highlight the differential effect environmental factors play in the progression to diabetes.

Incidence in Asians and Pacific Islanders

The SEARCH cohort provides the most detailed analysis of the incidence and prevalence of type 1 diabetes in Asians, Pacific Islanders, and mixed Asian/Pacific Islanders living in the United States. The estimated incidence rate was 6.4/100,000 for 0- to 9-year-olds and was 7.4/100,000 for 10- to 19-year-olds, much lower than that in other racial groups. The Asian subgroup had the lower rates of overweight and obesity among all racial backgrounds except non-Hispanic whites, whereas the Pacific Islanders subgroup had the highest rates.[26]

Seasonal variations in the incidence of type 1 diabetes

Type 1 diabetes incidence rates have been studied in relation to season of birth and season of onset, suggesting different periods of susceptibility coupled with the influence of environmental factors. Maternal, fetal, and childhood vitamin D levels, related to amount of ultraviolet light available and geographic location, are thought to influence immunity and metabolism at critical periods during development and contribute to the North–South difference in type 1 diabetes incidence.[35] Other environmental factors that have seasonal variations–such as viral infections–are thought to contribute to increased incidence rates later in life.

A large analysis of 19 regions included in the EURODIAB project failed to show an overall season of birth variation between seasons of birth in children younger than 15 years. The only statistically significant variation was found in several regions of United Kingdom, although there was no consistent pattern between these regions.[36]

In the United States, the SEARCH study found a lower risk of type 1 diabetes in children born between November and February. Children born in April to July had a highest risk of developing diabetes but only in some regions. Overall, it seemed children born in more northern states (Washington and Colorado) had a statistically significant risk ratio of developing diabetes depending on their birth month. Children from other SEARCH sites (Hawaii, South Carolina, and South California) did not have a statistically significant risk.[37]

The season of diagnosis seems to present as a more consistent pattern across different populations, with a generally accepted higher incidence rates in colder months. Data from 42 centers of the DIAMOND project showed a significant seasonal variation; 28 of these centers had peaks in the winter months (October to January) and 33 had peaks in the summer months (June to August). Overall, there was no consistent seasonal variation when adjusting for longitude, but centers farther away from the equator were more likely to have this type of variation. Also, children aged 5 to 14 were more likely to be subject to these variations than other age subgroups.[38]

Several US registries have analyzed seasonal variations. The Allegheny County registry found more cases diagnosed during the winter months (57%) compared with summer months (43%), but no statistically significant trend for their entire cohort between 1990 and 1994.[8]

Temporal trends

During the past century, type 1 diabetes in children has evolved form a rare, fatal condition before the discovery of insulin, to one of the most common chronic condition of this age group. Assessing the overall trend in incidence rate continues to be a daunting task, complicated by the inherent difference between populations and recording methods. More consistent registries have started in several areas in Europe and United States in the second half of the 20th century, but the past 20 years provide the most widespread data.[39]

The DIAMOND study reported an average increase in incidence among the 103 centers of 2.8% between 1990 and 1999, and an apparent acceleration as the average increase was 2.4% between 1990 and 1994 and 3.4% between 1995 and 1999. The increase in incidence varied among continents: 4.0% in Asia, 3.2% in Europe, 5.3% in North America, and a decrease of 3.6% in Central America and West Indies. The highest increase in incidence was seen in 0- to 4-year-olds (4.0%), followed by 5- to 9-year-olds (3.0%) and the 10- to 14-year-olds (2.1%). The increase in incidence was higher in areas with high or moderate overall incidence rate and more stable in centers with a low or very low incidence rate.[7]

The EURODIAB data, collected between 1989 and 2003, estimated an overall annual increase in incidence among the 20 registries under study of 3.9%, but the rates of increasing incidence varied between a 0.6% increase in Spain and a 9.3% increase in Poland. The highest increase in incidence was in children aged 0 to 4 years of age (5.4%), followed by 5- to 9-year-olds (4.3%). The lowest increase in incidence was in the 10- to 14-year-old group (2.9%). Further analysis of the European data showed an overall tendency toward a more rapid increase in incidence in girls aged 5 to 9 years old and slower in the 10- to 14-year-old age group than in boys.[12]

A follow-up report from the same European centers evaluating incidence of type 1 diabetes in children younger than 15 years of age during a 20-year period, between 1989 and 2008, showed a nonuniform increase in incidence rates, with periods of more or less rapid increase in various centers. The overall increase in the incidence rate remained between 3% and 4% per year. These suggest that environmental risk factors are changing over time in various ways across European countries.[40]

In the United States, the data collected by registries in different states during the past 30 years provide a similar nonuniform increase in incidence rates. The Philadelphia registry provides the most recent and consistent analysis of trends during the past 20 years for children aged 0 to 14 years. The incidence was relatively stable between 1985 and 1999 (13.4/100,000 between 1985 and 1989, 13.1/100,000 between 1990 and 1994, 14.8/100,000 between 1995 and 1999), but increased significantly to 16/100,000 per year between 2000 and 2004.[11]

The Allegheny County registry is the oldest one of its kind in United States, collecting data between 1965 and 1994, reported an overall stable incidence rate, but an interesting increase in black 0- to 19-year-olds between the first and the last cohort.[8] The Chicago Childhood Diabetes Registry reported similar incidence rates during 10 years of follow-up: 10.4/100,000 per year between 1994 and 1998 and 11.2/100,000 per year between 1999 and 2003.[9] In Colorado, 2 registries collected data spanning 27 years on the incidence of type 1 diabetes in children aged 0 to 17 years. The Colorado IDDM Study Registry collected data between 1978 and 1988 and reported an overall incidence rate of 14.8/100,000 per year. As a member of the SEARCH study–and using different ascertainment methodology, the incidence was analyzed in the same region and age group between 2002 and 2004 and reported an annual incidence rate of 23.9/100,000, corresponding to an increase in incidence of 2.3% per year.[25]

RISK FACTORS

The cause of type 1 diabetes is multifactorial and incompletely understood. The current model holds that type 1 diabetes arises in genetically susceptible children exposed to environmental triggers.

Genetics

Genotype is an important role in the development of type 1 diabetes. The lifetime risk of developing type 1 diabetes in the general population is approximately 0.4%, and this risk increases significantly with a first-degree relative with type 1 diabetes.[41] Siblings have a 3% to 6% risk of developing type 1 diabetes and children have a 1% to 2% risk if the mother has type 1 diabetes and a 3% to 5% risk if the father has type 1 diabetes.[42] Siblings of children with type 1 diabetes diagnosed before age 7 years have the highest risk. Twin studies provide further evidence of genetic risk in type 1 diabetes. In a large study of twin pairs in Finland, the concordance rates for type 1 diabetes were 27.3% in monozygotic twins and 3.8% in dizygotic twins.[43] The risk of type 1 diabetes increased with younger age of onset in the index twin.

In the 1970s, type 1 diabetes was recognized as being associated with genetic variants in the human leukocyte antigen (HLA) on chromosome 6p21.3.[44,45] HLA class II DR4 and DR3 are most closely associated with type 1 diabetes, and the combination of the 2 alleles, DR3/DR4, produces the highest genetic susceptibility.[46] Those children with the highest risk genotype have a 5% risk of getting diabetes by age 15 years.[47] HLA variants account for approximately 50% of type 1 diabetes genetic susceptibility. More than 40 genes account for the remaining 50% genetic risk.[48] After the HLA alleles, polymorphisms in INS (encoding proinsulin) and PTPN22 (involved in T-cell regulation) contribute the most genetic risk for type 1 diabetes.[49,50]

Several studies have demonstrated that more cases of type 1 diabetes are occurring in children with lower-risk HLA genotypes.[51,52] This suggests that the increasing incidence may be driven by environmental factors.

Environmental Factors

The role of environmental risk factors in the development of type 1 diabetes is suggested by the modest concordance rates between twins and studies of migrant populations. Studies have demonstrated that being born in a high-incidence country increases the risk of type 1 diabetes in children of parents who have migrated from low-incidence regions.[53,54] Furthermore, higher socioeconomic status is associated with increased type 1 diabetes risk in the SEARCH cohort.[55] This finding concurs with a European study demonstrating that type 1 diabetes incidence correlates with indicators of national prosperity, such as gross national product and infant mortality.[56] This correlation is behind the hygiene hypothesis, which proposes that improved living standards and decreased infectious burden drive the increase in autoimmune diseases in industrialized countries.[57]

Numerous environmental factors have been proposed and investigated, mainly in case-control studies. Given the seasonal variation in type 1 diabetes occurrence, a viral trigger has been long sought with enteroviruses being the main candidate.[58] In a Finnish study, children who developed diabetes-associated autoantibodies had higher levels of enterovirus antibodies than did control subjects.[59] Additionally, enteroviral RNA has been found in the pancreas of patients with type 1 diabetes at autopsy and children who died of acute enteroviral infections.[60,61] However, a decreased incidence of enterovirus infections during the period of increasing type 1 diabetes incidence refutes the role of this virus in type 1 diabetes pathogenesis. The Philadelphia registry demonstrated an epidemic of type 1 diabetes in 1993, 2 years after a measles epidemic.[29] Other viruses studied, including mumps, measles, cytomegalovirus, and retroviruses, have not provided a convincing link to type 1 diabetes.[58]

Dietary factors have been extensively studied without conclusive and consistent findings. Early exposure to cow's milk protein has been linked with increased type 1 diabetes risk.[62] A cow's milk protein, bovine serum albumin, shares a structurally homologous sequence with an islet cell antigen, which suggests molecular mimicry as the trigger for β-cell destruction.[63] The ongoing Trial to Reduce Insulin-dependent Diabetes Mellitus in the Genetically at Risk (TRIGR) aims to identify whether delaying exposure to cow's milk protein reduces the risk of type 1 diabetes in genetically at-risk children.[64] In the initial pilot study, weaning to an extensively hydrolyzed formula significantly decreased the cumulative incidence of diabetes auto-antibodies. However, the Diabetes Autoimmunity Study in the Young (DAISY) in the United States, a prospective study of children at high genetic risk of developing type 1 diabetes, found no association between early exposure to cow's milk and β-cell autoimmunity.[65]

The role of vitamin D has also been studied without conclusive findings. Lower levels of 25-OH vitamin D have been reported in new diagnosed cases of type 1 diabetes compared with controls, and increased maternal intake of vitamin D is associated with decreased risk of diabetes autoantibodies in offspring.[66,67] However, as with cow's milk protein, the DAISY study found no association between vitamin D levels or intake and the development of diabetes autoantibodies or progression to type 1 diabetes.[68]

A more recently identified and controversial risk factor for type 1 diabetes is obesity. The accelerator hypothesis postulates that the increase in type 1 diabetes is related to earlier disease onset driven by weight-related insulin resistance.[69] In genetically susceptible individuals, insulin resistance drives both β-cell apoptosis and the immune response, leading to type 1 diabetes.[70] The rise in type 1 diabetes concurrent with the rise in obesity and type 2 diabetes lends support to this theory. However, studies relating age of type 1 diabetes presentation with weight or body mass index have found conflicting results.[69,71]

The risk factors for the development of type 1 diabetes in children remain incompletely understood. Genotype plays a significant but small role in type 1 diabetes risk. Studies of environmental factors, ranging from viruses to obesity, have found conflicting results with no clear trigger identified.

SUMMARY

The incidence of type 1 diabetes in children has been increasing by approximately 3% per year worldwide, particularly in children younger than age 5. Evidence of an increase in incidence and data related to epidemics have left unanswered questions about etiologic factors. Large-scale registry consortiums, particularly in Europe, have provided the most comprehensive data related to type 1 diabetes in youth, yet systematic surveillance is still lacking. It would be far more effective to develop a national system of surveillance similar to cancer prototype—mandating case reporting of diabetes—so that the global rising incidence of type 1 diabetes, and the search for environmental risk factors, can be addressed with a worldwide collaborative approach.

REFERENCES

1. National Center for Health Statistics, Centers for Disease Control and Prevention. 2007-2009. National Health Interview Survey (NHIS). Available at: http://www.cdc. gov/nchs/nhis.htm. Accessed July 21, 2012.
2. Tao B, Pietropaolo M, Atkinson M, et al. Estimating the cost of type 1 diabetes in the U.S.: a propensity score matching method. PLoS One 2010;5:e11501.
3. Maahs DM, West NA, Lawrence JM, et al. Epidemiology of type 1 diabetes. Endocrinol Metab Clin North Am 2010;39:481–97.
4. Diabetes Epidemiology Research International Group. Geographic patterns of childhood insulin-dependent diabetes mellitus. Diabetes 1988;37:1113–9.
5. WHO Diamond Project Group. WHO multinational project for childhood diabetes. Diabetes Care 1990;13:1062–8.
6. LaPorte R, Matsushima M, Chang Y. Prevalence and incidence of insulin-dependent diabetes. In: Maureen I, Harris, editors. Diabetes in America. 2nd edition. Washington, DC: National Institutes of Health, NIDDK; 1995. p. 37–46.
7. DIAMOND Project Group. Incidence and trends of childhood type 1 diabetes worldwide 1990-1999. Diabet Med 2006;23:857–66.
8. Libman IM, LaPorte RE, Becker D, et al. Was there an epidemic of diabetes in nonwhite adolescents in Allegheny County, Pennsylvania? Diabetes Care 1998; 21:1278–81.
9. Smith TL, Drum ML, Lipton RB. Incidence of childhood type I and non-type 1 diabetes mellitus in a diverse population: the Chicago Childhood Diabetes Registry, 1994 to 2003. J Pediatr Endocrinol Metab 2007;20:1093–107.
10. Dabelea D, Bell RA, D'Agostino RB Jr, et al. Incidence of diabetes in youth in the United States. JAMA 2007;297:2716–24.
11. Lipman, TH, Levitt Katz, LE, Aguilar, A, et al. The epidemiology of type 1 and type 2 diabetes in youth in Philadelphia: 2000-2004. In 69th Annual Meeting of the American Diabetes Association. New Orleans, LA: Diabetes 2009;58:288–OR.
12. Patterson CC, Dahlquist GG, Gyurus E, et al. Incidence trends for childhood type 1 diabetes in Europe during 1989-2003 and predicted new cases 2005-20: a multicentre prospective registration study. Lancet 2009;373:2027–33.
13. Diabetes in the young in International Diabetes Federation. IDF Diabetes Atlas. 5th edition. Brussels, Belgium: International Diabetes federation; 2011.http:// www.idf.org/diabetesatlas. Accessed July 21, 2012.
14. Liese AD, D'Agostino RB Jr, Hamman RF, et al. The burden of diabetes mellitus among US youth: prevalence estimates from the SEARCH for Diabetes in Youth Study. Pediatrics 2006;118:1510–8.
15. Lipman TH, Minakmami J, Hughes J, et al. Population based survey of the prevalence of type 1 and type 2 diabetes in school children in Philadelphia. Diabetes 2006;55:A219.
16. Sardu C, Cocco E, Mereu A, et al. Population-based study of 12 autoimmune diseases in Sardinia, Italy: prevalence and comorbidity. PLoS One 2012;7:e32487.
17. Blanchard JF, Dean H, Anderson K, et al. Incidence and prevalence of diabetes in children aged 0-14 years in Manitoba, Canada, 1985-1993. Diabetes Care 1997;20:512–5.
18. Al-Herbish AS, El-Mouzan MI, Al-Salloum AA, et al. Prevalence of type 1 diabetes mellitus in Saudi Arabian children and adolescents. Saudi Med J 2008;29: 1285–8.
19. Akesen E, Turan S, Guran T, et al. Prevalence of type 1 diabetes mellitus in 6-18-yr-old school children living in Istanbul, Turkey. Pediatr Diabetes 2011;12:567–71.

20. Mayer-Davis EJ, Bell RA, Dabelea D, et al. The many faces of diabetes in American youth: type 1 and type 2 diabetes in five race and ethnic populations: the SEARCH for Diabetes in Youth Study. Diabetes Care 2009;32(Suppl 2):S99–101.
21. Liese AD, Lawson A, Song HR, et al. Evaluating geographic variation in type 1 and type 2 diabetes mellitus incidence in youth in four US regions. Health Place 2010;16:547–56.
22. Casu A, Pascutto C, Bernardinelli L, et al. Type 1 diabetes among Sardinian children is increasing: the Sardinian diabetes register for children aged 0-14 years (1989-1999). Diabetes Care 2004;27:1623–9.
23. Harjutsalo V, Sjoberg L, Tuomilehto J. Time trends in the incidence of type 1 diabetes in Finnish children: a cohort study. Lancet 2008;371:1777–82.
24. Derraik JG, Reed PW, Jefferies C, et al. Increasing incidence and age at diagnosis among children with type 1 diabetes mellitus over a 20-year period in Auckland (New Zealand). PLoS One 2012;7:e32640.
25. Vehik K, Hamman RF, Lezotte D, et al. Increasing incidence of type 1 diabetes in 0- to 17-year-old Colorado youth. Diabetes Care 2007;30:503–9.
26. Mayer-Davis EJ, Beyer J, Bell RA, et al. Diabetes in African American youth: prevalence, incidence, and clinical characteristics: the SEARCH for Diabetes in Youth Study. Diabetes Care 2009;32(Suppl 2):S112–22.
27. Dokheel TM. An epidemic of childhood diabetes in the United States? Evidence from Allegheny County, Pennsylvania. Pittsburgh Diabetes Epidemiology Research Group. Diabetes Care 1993;16:1606–11.
28. LaPorte RE, Fishbein HA, Drash AL, et al. The Pittsburgh Insulin-Dependent Diabetes Mellitus (IDDM) registry. The incidence of insulin-dependent diabetes mellitus in Allegheny County, Pennsylvania (1965-1976). Diabetes 1981;30:279–84.
29. Lipman TH, Chang Y, Murphy KM. The epidemiology of type 1 diabetes in children in Philadelphia 1990-1994: evidence of an epidemic. Diabetes Care 2002;25:1969–75.
30. Lipman TH, Jawad AF, Murphy KM, et al. Incidence of type 1 diabetes in Philadelphia is higher in black than white children from 1995 to 1999: epidemic or misclassification? Diabetes Care 2006;29:2391–5.
31. Lorenzi M, Cagliero E, Schmidt NJ. Racial differences in incidence of juvenile-onset type 1 diabetes: epidemiologic studies in southern California. Diabetologia 1985;28:734–8.
32. Lipman TH. The epidemiology of type I diabetes in children 0-14 yr of age in Philadelphia. Diabetes Care 1993;16:922–5.
33. Frazer de Llado TE, Gonzalez de Pijem L, Hawk B. Incidence of IDDM in children living in Puerto Rico. Puerto Rican IDDM Coalition. Diabetes Care 1998;21:744–6.
34. Lawrence JM, Mayer-Davis EJ, Reynolds K, et al. Diabetes in Hispanic American youth: prevalence, incidence, demographics, and clinical characteristics: the SEARCH for Diabetes in Youth Study. Diabetes Care 2009;32(Suppl 2):S123–32.
35. Luong K, Nguyen LT, Nguyen DN. The role of vitamin D in protecting type 1 diabetes mellitus. Diabetes Metab Res Rev 2005;21:338–46.
36. McKinney PA. Seasonality of birth in patients with childhood type I diabetes in 19 European regions. Diabetologia 2001;44(Suppl 3):B67–74.
37. Kahn HS, Morgan TM, Case LD, et al. Association of type 1 diabetes with month of birth among U.S. youth: the SEARCH for Diabetes in Youth Study. Diabet Care 2009;32:2010–5.
38. Moltchanova EV, Schreier N, Lammi N, et al. Seasonal variation of diagnosis of type 1 diabetes mellitus in children worldwide. Diabet Med 2009;26:673–8.

39. Gale EA. The rise of childhood type 1 diabetes in the 20th century. Diabetes 2002;51:3353–61.
40. Patterson CC, Gyurus E, Rosenbauer J, et al. Trends in childhood type 1 diabetes incidence in Europe during 1989-2008: evidence of non-uniformity over time in rates of increase. Diabetologia 2012;55(8):2142–7 [Epub 2012 May 26].
41. Mehers KL, Gillespie KM. The genetic basis for type 1 diabetes. Br Med Bull 2008;88:115–29.
42. Steck AK, Barriga KJ, Emery LM, et al. Secondary attack rate of type 1 diabetes in Colorado families. Diabet Care 2005;28:296–300.
43. Hyttinen V, Kaprio J, Kinnunen L, et al. Genetic liability of type 1 diabetes and the onset age among 22,650 young Finnish twin pairs: a nationwide follow-up study. Diabetes 2003;52:1052–5.
44. Singal DP, Blajchman MA. Histocompatibility (HL-A) antigens, lymphocytotoxic antibodies and tissue antibodies in patients with diabetes mellitus. Diabetes 1973;22:429–32.
45. Cudworth AG, Woodrow JC. Evidence for HL-A-linked genes in "juvenile" diabetes mellitus. Br Med J 1975;3:133–5.
46. Todd JA, Bell JI, McDevitt HO. HLA-DQ beta gene contributes to susceptibility and resistance to insulin-dependent diabetes mellitus. Nature 1987;329:599–604.
47. Lambert AP, Gillespie KM, Thomson G, et al. Absolute risk of childhood-onset type 1 diabetes defined by human leukocyte antigen class II genotype: a population-based study in the United Kingdom. J Clin Endocrinol Metab 2004;89:4037–43.
48. Steck AK, Rewers MJ. Genetics of type 1 diabetes. Clin Chem 2011;57:176–85.
49. Bell GI, Horita S, Karam JH. A polymorphic locus near the human insulin gene is associated with insulin-dependent diabetes mellitus. Diabetes 1984;33:176–83.
50. Bottini N, Musumeci L, Alonso A, et al. A functional variant of lymphoid tyrosine phosphatase is associated with type I diabetes. Nat Genet 2004;36:337–8.
51. Gillespie KM, Bain SC, Barnett AH, et al. The rising incidence of childhood type 1 diabetes and reduced contribution of high-risk HLA haplotypes. Lancet 2004;364:1699–700.
52. Fourlanos S, Varney MD, Tait BD, et al. The rising incidence of type 1 diabetes is accounted for by cases with lower-risk human leukocyte antigen genotypes. Diabetes Care 2008;31:1546–9.
53. Soderstrom U, Aman J, Hjern A. Being born in Sweden increases the risk for type 1 diabetes - a study of migration of children to Sweden as a natural experiment. Acta Paediatr 2012;101:73–7.
54. Raymond NT, Jones JR, Swift PG, et al. Comparative incidence of type I diabetes in children aged under 15 years from South Asian and white or other ethnic backgrounds in Leicestershire, UK, 1989 to 1998. Diabetologia 2001;44(Suppl 3):B32–6.
55. Liese AD, Puett RC, Lamichhane AP, et al. Neighborhood level risk factors for type 1 diabetes in youth: the SEARCH case-control study. Int J Health Geogr 2012;11:1.
56. Patterson CC, Dahlquist G, Soltesz G, et al. Is childhood-onset type I diabetes a wealth-related disease? An ecological analysis of European incidence rates. Diabetologia 2001;44(Suppl 3):B9–16.
57. Okada H, Kuhn C, Feillet H, et al. The 'hygiene hypothesis' for autoimmune and allergic diseases: an update. Clin Exp Immunol 2010;160:1–9.
58. Roivainen M, Klingel K. Virus infections and type 1 diabetes risk. Curr Diab Rep 2010;10:350–6.

59. Sadeharju K, Lonnrot M, Kimpimaki T, et al. Enterovirus antibody levels during the first two years of life in prediabetic autoantibody-positive children. Diabetologia 2001;44:818–23.

60. Ylipaasto P, Klingel K, Lindberg AM, et al. Enterovirus infection in human pancreatic islet cells, islet tropism in vivo and receptor involvement in cultured islet beta cells. Diabetologia 2004;47:225–39.

61. Dotta F, Censini S, van Halteren AG, et al. Coxsackie B4 virus infection of beta cells and natural killer cell insulitis in recent-onset type 1 diabetic patients. Proc Natl Acad Sci U S A 2007;104:5115–20.

62. Virtanen SM, Rasanen L, Ylonen K, et al. Early introduction of dairy products associated with increased risk of IDDM in Finnish children. The Childhood in Diabetes in Finland Study Group. Diabetes 1993;42:1786–90.

63. Miyazaki I, Cheung RK, Gaedigk R, et al. T cell activation and anergy to islet cell antigen in type I diabetes. J Immunol 1995;154:1461–9.

64. Knip M, Virtanen SM, Becker D, et al. Early feeding and risk of type 1 diabetes: experiences from the Trial to Reduce Insulin-dependent diabetes mellitus in the Genetically at Risk (TRIGR). Am J Clin Nutr 2011;94:1814S–20S.

65. Norris JM, Beaty B, Klingensmith G, et al. Lack of association between early exposure to cow's milk protein and beta-cell autoimmunity. Diabetes Autoimmunity Study in the Young (DAISY). JAMA 1996;276:609–14.

66. Pozzilli P, Manfrini S, Crino A, et al. Low levels of 25-hydroxyvitamin D3 and 1,25-dihydroxyvitamin D3 in patients with newly diagnosed type 1 diabetes. Horm Metab Res 2005;37:680–3.

67. Fronczak CM, Baron AE, Chase HP, et al. In utero dietary exposures and risk of islet autoimmunity in children. Diabetes Care 2003;26:3237–42.

68. Simpson M, Brady H, Yin X, et al. No association of vitamin D intake or 25-hydroxyvitamin D levels in childhood with risk of islet autoimmunity and type 1 diabetes: the Diabetes Autoimmunity Study in the Young (DAISY). Diabetologia 2011;54:2779–88.

69. Kibirige M, Metcalf B, Renuka R, et al. Testing the accelerator hypothesis: the relationship between body mass and age at diagnosis of type 1 diabetes. Diabetes Care 2003;26:2865–70.

70. Wilkin TJ. The accelerator hypothesis: weight gain as the missing link between type I and type II diabetes. Diabetologia 2001;44:914–22.

71. O'Connell MA, Donath S, Cameron FJ. Major increase in type 1 diabetes: no support for the accelerator hypothesis. Diabet Med 2007;24:920–3.

Update on Global Intervention Studies in Type 1 Diabetes

Jane L. Chiang, MD[a],*, Michael J. Haller, MD[b],
Desmond A. Schatz, MD[b]

KEYWORDS

- Type 1 diabetes • Intervention • Prevention • Combination therapy

KEY POINTS

- Intervention studies target individuals shortly after disease onset, seeking to preserve residual β-cell function and maintain normoglycemia while also decreasing both hypoglycemia and long-term complications.
- Prevention studies seek to halt autoimmune destruction and prevent clinical onset of type 1 diabetes (T1D) in at-risk individuals.
- Currently, approaches to reverse or prevent T1D remains elusive.

INTRODUCTION

A key challenge in developing an interdiction strategy for type 1 diabetes (T1D) is knowing precisely where to focus the effort, namely, intervention versus prevention. Intervention studies target individuals shortly after disease onset, seeking to preserve residual β-cell function and maintain normoglycemia while decreasing both hypoglycemia and long-term complications. Prevention studies seek to halt autoimmune destruction and prevent clinical onset of T1D in at-risk individuals.[1] Prevention studies may be further divided into primary prevention (prevention of autoimmunity) and secondary prevention (prevention of overt hyperglycemia in individuals with established autoimmunity). Because T1D is a devastating disease primarily striking children, searching for a therapy with the ideal balance of efficacy and safety is crucial. The initial "cure" may be an imperfect agent with either suboptimal preservation abilities and/or significant adverse effects. However, the attributes of any therapy may or may not outweigh the burdens associated with the natural progression of T1D and daily diabetes management.

Despite ongoing debate regarding optimal study design, acting early (ie, primary prevention) likely represents the best opportunity for effectively eradicating T1D.

[a] Division of Endocrinology, Department of Pediatrics, Stanford University, 300 Pasteur Drive, G 313, Stanford, CA 94305, USA; [b] Division of Endocrinology, Department of Pediatrics, University of Florida, PO Box 100296, Gainesville, FL 32610, USA
* Corresponding author.
E-mail address: jane.chiang0@gmail.com

Endocrinol Metab Clin N Am 41 (2012) 695–712
http://dx.doi.org/10.1016/j.ecl.2012.07.003
0889-8529/12/$ – see front matter © 2012 Elsevier Inc. All rights reserved.

Although prevention studies will likely be more effective and require less aggressive therapies than intervention, accurately predicting disease is challenging. Furthermore, early prevention therapies must be extremely safe as they would be administered to people who may never actually develop T1D. In addition, many of the subjects will be the most vulnerable population: young children. Over time, disease identification becomes easier as at-risk individuals manifest autoimmune markers. Ironically, as prediction of disease becomes more accurate, the chance to effectively intervene may be lost because extensive β-cell destruction may have already occurred **Fig. 1**.

Identifying eligible subjects requires screening thousands of individuals only to isolate the very small minority who develop the disease. Clinical trials evaluating prevention require multicenter and multinational collaboration and, thus, are expensive and labor-intensive. Were one to eliminate screening and move to a model of universal prevention, the difficulties of screening would be markedly reduced, but concerns over equipoise would, once again, be raised to levels beyond those in which individuals at elevated risk are identified and subjected to intervention.[2]

In contrast to prevention studies, intervention studies with newly diagnosed T1D patients have fewer barriers, primarily because there is no need to identify subjects. Autoimmune markers confirm the presence of T1D and, because the diagnosis of clinical diabetes has already been made, subjects are often more interested in participating in a clinical trial. Therefore, given the limited β-cell mass and the presence of established autoimmunity, the key to designing interdiction efforts lays in finding an acceptable balance between potential efficacy and safety: a physician needs to intervene at an early enough stage with an effective, but safe, therapy. Low-risk therapies can ethically be tested in prevention studies, but require a large number of individuals, are costly, and may take years to document a successful outcome. On the other hand, high-risk therapies are used in intervention studies in which the target population is smaller (ie, those with T1D vs those at risk of developing T1D) and may require a shorter time to document potential efficacy. To ascertain equipoise between risk and benefit, agents with potentially significant side effects (eg, immunomodulatory

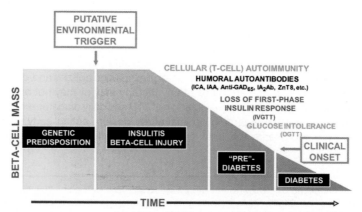

Fig. 1. Treatment dilemma for T1D. Animal models suggest that an earlier intervention is more effective and often requires less aggressive strategies. Identifying such individuals is often difficult and time-consuming. Markers associated with disease onset (eg, autoimmune markers) facilitate later interventions. However, these therapies are more aggressive and are often associated with safety issues. (*From* Skyler JS, Ricordi C. Stopping type 1 diabetes: attempts to prevent or cure type 1 diabetes in man. Diabetes 2011;60:2; with permission.)

and immunosuppressive therapies) have currently been used in intervention studies in recent onset patients, whereas prevention studies use lower-risk therapies that apply to broader populations.

In recent decades, numerous agents have been explored as possibilities to cure or prevent T1D. Sadly, drug toxicities and limited magnitude and duration of efficacy have resulted in limited enthusiasm for many previously promising therapies. Due to space constraints, this article highlights only the key therapeutics that have elucidated understanding of the disease.

PREVENTION STRATEGIES

The ultimate goal is to eradicate T1D. Insight into pre-T1D has enabled efforts to identify and potentially prevent the disease in those at risk. Because memory is fundamental to the immune system, it is unlikely that a cure will emerge without being able to prevent the disease from reoccurring. Subjects can now be stratified according to their risk profile. Data from the Diabetes Prevention Trial-Type 1 (DPT-1) have identified characteristics of individuals in the highest-risk cohort, specifically those with abnormal glucose tolerance who are autoantibody-positive relatives of T1D patients. These individuals have a rapid rate of disease progression, with a greater than 75% risk of developing T1D over 5 years.[3] Because the likelihood of T1D development is so high, these study subjects might reasonably be exposed to a therapeutic with a slightly higher risk: benefit profile.

In that regard, patients in this very high risk group are now being enrolled in a TrialNet study using teplizumab (anti-CD3) in a single 14-day course of the drug with the aim of delaying or preventing diabetes onset (National Clinical Trial [NCT]01030861). The primary outcome measure is T1D development as defined by the American Diabetes Association and based on glucose testing or presence of unequivocal hyperglycemia with acute metabolic decompensation. Several additional secondary prevention trials are enrolling relatives at lower risk for T1D (see later discussion).

Insulin

Insulin is believed to be an early and primary autoantigen in T1D. Studies in the non-obese diabetic (NOD) mouse[4] and pilot human studies demonstrated that early exposure to oral insulin was effective in preventing diabetes and may induce immune tolerance. DPT-1 (NCT00004984) sought to determine if the immunomodulatory effects of recurrent insulin exposure, subcutaneous or oral, could prevent or delay T1D onset. DPT-1 was one of the first large multicenter, randomized, placebo-controlled trials to strive for T1D prevention. A massive screening effort yielded 3500 individuals with islet cell cytoplasmic autoantibody plus or minus insulin autoantibody (IAA) positive from a screening of over 100,000 first and second-degree relatives of T1D patients. Of these, 339 enrolled in the parenteral arm and 372 in the oral insulin arm. Both forms of insulin proved safe, but neither oral nor subcutaneous insulin demonstrated efficacy.[5] Interestingly, a post hoc observation of the DPT-1 data demonstrated that at-risk patients, with higher IAA titers (>80 nU/mL) and who received oral insulin, experienced a 5 to 10 year delay in the onset of disease, an effect that was sustained even after cessation of the oral insulin therapy.[6] To facilitate future studies, a multicentered consortium funded primarily by the National Institutes of Health, TrialNet, was created. TrialNet is currently recruiting a for a follow-up study to determine if oral insulin can indeed delay T1D onset in those intermediate risk individuals with two or more islet autoantibodies, including IAA (NCT00419562). Almost 20,000 relatives are being screened annually through the TrialNet Pathway to

Prevention study, but ongoing efforts are required to ensure that the large number of subjects needed for these prevention trials can be efficiently identified (NCT00097292).

The Finnish Diabetes Prediction and Prevention Project sought to use intranasal insulin in very young genetically at-risk autoantibody positive subjects. Intranasal insulin proved to be safe but ineffective (NCT00223613).[6] The Australian Intranasal Insulin Trial (INIT) I, a safety study performed in adults, confirmed that exposure to intranasal insulin caused immune changes consistent with mucosal tolerance to insulin, potentially causing insulin to act like a vaccine.[7] INIT II is evaluating the efficacy of a higher dose of intranasal insulin (440 IU insulin daily for 7 days then weekly for 12 months, and includes older subjects, ages 4–30 years). The study aim is to determine if intranasal insulin can prevent β-cell destruction in at-risk individuals (NCT00336674). In patients with latent autoimmune diabetes in adults, nasal insulin was associated with a decreased T-cell response, suggesting that there may be an immunologic effect of intranasal insulin that merits further investigation.[8]

The aim of the Primary Intervention with Oral Insulin for the Prevention of T1D Trial (Pre-POINT) study is to evaluate if insulin can delay or even prevent autoimmunity and T1D.[9] The preventative treatment with oral insulin is intended to induce tolerance in children with high genetic risk (www.diabetes-point.org). Another study using insulin B-chain immunotherapy in newly diagnosed T1D patients demonstrated specific T-cell responses to nonmetabolically active insulin but no effect on C-peptide, when compared with placebo.[10]

Glutamic Acid Decarboxylase 65

Glutamic acid decarboxylase 65 (GAD65) was another potential autoantigen targeted for therapeutic use in T1D. Data from NOD mice[11] have shown that GAD65 vaccination may prevent T1D development. GAD65 (Diamyd) dosing (20 μg) in a small study of adults with latent autoimmune diabetes demonstrated no adverse events and preservation of endogenous β-cell function versus placebo (PubMed–indexed for MEDLINE:15993359). This was an intervention study. A phase II trial involving 70 children (10–18 years) with T1D, demonstrated β-cell preservation with no treatment-related adverse events.[12] However, a phase III study in 334 subjects (ages 10–20 years, diagnosed within 3 months) with GAD-alum therapy versus placebo failed to demonstrate β-cell preservation, based on C-peptide level from baseline to 15 months. The proportion of any adverse or serious adverse events was the same in the treatment and placebo group[13] (NCT00723411). No prevention studies have yet been done.

INTERVENTION STRATEGIES

In contrast to antigen-specific efforts in prevention trials, intervention trials have largely focused on targeting the immune system to halt β-cell destruction.[14–17] In general, interventional approaches have focused on three broad areas: antigen-specific therapies (eg, insulin, GAD), immunosuppressants, and immunomodulators.[1] Although many of these agents have demonstrated preliminary C-peptide preservation in clinical trials, many agents have been abandoned owing of intolerable associated toxicities (eg, nephrotoxicity for cyclosporine). As a result of experiences with higher risk therapies, several low-risk therapies, such as nicotinamide,[18] ketotifen,[19] Bacille Calmette-Guerin,[20] and autologous cord blood infusion[21] were explored. Although safe, these approaches failed to preserve β-cell function. Additional low-risk non–antigen-specific therapies, such as alpha-1 antitrypsin,[22] heat shock protein-derived DiaPep227,[23] and avoidance of cow milk proteins[24] (prevention study), are currently under investigation **Fig. 2**.

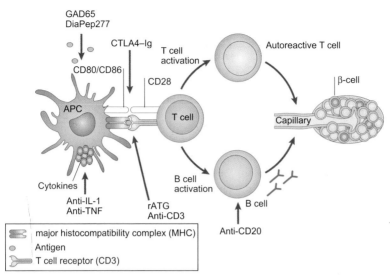

Fig. 2. Postulated mechanism of action in T1D. The exact mechanism of action for how T1D occurs is not clear. Speculations on the current role of antigens, antigen presenting cells, cytokines, T and B cells and their effects on the β cell are presented here. (*From* Waldron-Lynch F, Herold KC. Immunomodulatory therapy to preserve pancreatic b-cell function in T1D. Nat Rev Drug Discov 2011;10:439–52. Reprinted by permission from Macmillan Publishers Ltd.)

DiaPep227

Heat-shock protein (hsp60) is a known self-antigen. An immunomodulatory peptide from hsp60, p277, arrested β-cell destruction and maintained insulin production in newly diabetic NOD mice. A phase II study of DiaPep277 treatment seemed to preserve endogenous insulin production in newly diagnosed (<6 months) T1D adults, perhaps through induction of a shift from T-helper-1 to T-helper-2 cytokines produced by the autoimmune T cells.[25] A phase III trial is currently ongoing in recent onset adults with T1D (NCT01103284).

Anti-CD3

T1D is believed to result from T-cell–mediated destruction of pancreatic β cells. Potentially removing such autoreactive T cells using monoclonal antibodies to CD3 could, therefore, prevent and even reverse diabetes.[26,27] Anti-CD3 was first used to prevent rejection in organ transplant recipients. Humanized anti-CD3 antibodies, hOKT3gl (Ala-Ala/Teplizumab) (NCT00378508), and ChAglyCD3 (TRX4/Otelixizumab) (NCT00451321), were developed to induce "tolerance" to self by eliminating autoreactive T cells and potentially increasing selective regulatory T cells. The latter are hypothesized to enhance tolerance and counteract the effector T cells responsible for destroying β cells. Initial studies conducted in T1D patients showed promising results with long-term (eg, 18–24 months posttherapy) preservation of C-peptide.[28,29] Exploratory findings from the Phase III Protégé study (subjects diagnosed with T1D ≤12 weeks, n = 513, ages 8–35 years) suggest that teplizumab may prevent decline in β-cell function, as measured by C-peptide. The subjects were randomized to receive teplizumab for 14-days full-dose, 14-day low-dose, 6-day full-dose, or placebo (NCT00385697). The primary composite outcome was the percentage of patients with insulin use of less than 0.5 U/kg per day and hemoglobin A1c (HbA1c) of less than 6.5% at 1 year, but did not differ between the groups at 1 year. Five percent (19 out of 415) of patients in the teplizumab groups were not taking insulin at 1 year, compared with no patients in the placebo group at 1 year ($P = .03$).[30]

The Phase III DEFEND-1 study, evaluating ChAglyCD3 (TRX4/otelixizumab), studied the effect of humanized anti-CD3 antibodies on β-cell preservation in recent onset (≤3 months of T1D diagnosis) (NCT00678886). Unfortunately, DEFEND-1 did not meet the primary efficacy endpoint (change in C-peptide at month 12). DEFEND-2 (NCT01123083), a confirmatory Phase III, has been suspended pending review of the DEFEND-1 results[31] (http://us.gsk.com).

Anti-CD20

T cells have traditionally been implicated as the primary effector cells in T1D. However, recent evidence suggests that B cells may also play a role.[32] Rituximab (Rituxan), an anti-CD20 monoclonal antibody, downregulates B lymphocyte signaling of T cells and, therefore, may inhibit cytotoxic T cells in triggering islet injury. Rituximab is a potent immunosuppressant used for treatment of autoimmune non-Hodgkin lymphoma, chronic lymphocytic leukemia, and rheumatoid arthritis (www.fda.gov; www.rituxan.com). Preclinical data with anti-B-lymphocyte activities demonstrated efficacy in preventing and reversing diabetes in the NOD mouse.[33,34] A Phase II TrialNet study evaluated rituximab in new-onset T1D patients (n = 87, ages 8–40 years, ≤100 days of diagnosis) in a randomized, placebo controlled trial to determine if four weekly IV infusions safely preserve C-peptide. One-year outcome data showed that four doses of rituximab partially preserved C-peptide in those with T1D (mean area under the curve (AUC) c-peptide 0.56 pmol/mL vs 0.47 pmol/mL with placebo) making the mean level for the treatment group 20% higher than that for placebo ($P = .03$). The results were similar at 4 hours ($P = .009$) and among the 71 patients who received all four infusions ($P = .004$).[32] (NCT00279305) In addition, the rituximab group had significantly lower levels of HbA1C and required less insulin.

Patients receiving rituximab did experience adverse events, mostly grade 1 or grade 2, especially after the first infusion. The reactions occurred less frequently with subsequent rituximab infusions, and there was no increase in infections or neutropenia. CD19+ B lymphocytes were depleted in patients with rituximab, but levels increased to 69% of baseline values at 1 year. B-cell involvement in a presumed T-cell–mediated disease confirms the complexity of this autoimmune disorder. Although the rituximab study did demonstrate that anti-CD20 intervention statistically preserves C-peptide more effectively than placebo, we must remind ourselves that statistical significance does not always equate to clinical relevance. As such, even significant studies must be considered in terms of their capacity to impact patients' lives when debating equipoise.

Mycofenolate Mofetil and Anti-CD25

Investigators surmised that using two agents with different mechanisms of action could improve efficacy while limiting toxicity. The combination of mycofenolate mofetil (MMF) (immunosuppressant) and the anti-CD25 antibody, daclizumab (DZB), involved a single IV infusion of DZB with daily oral MMF administered to new-onset T1D subjects. Unfortunately, neither MMF-alone nor MMF in combination with DZB had an effect on the loss of C-peptide in subjects with new onset T1D (NCT00100178).[35]

Cytotoxic T-Lymphocyte Antigen-4 Immunoglobulin

Cytotoxic T-Lymphocyte Antigen-4 (CTLA-4) inhibits an important stimulatory pathway in the activation of T cells. It is thought to arrest or slow T-cell–mediated autoimmune destruction of β cells and preserve their function. It is expressed on the surface of T-helper cells and transmits an inhibitory signal to T cells by blocking the stimulatory effect of CD28 binding.[36,37] CTLA-4 may also impact tolerance-inducing regulatory T cells. It has received Food and Drug Administration (FDA) approval for rheumatoid arthritis (Abatacept/Orencia), and is now being explored for its potential use in T1D. The TrialNet consortium is completing a Phase II randomized, double-blind, placebo controlled trial of CTLA-4-Ig/placebo in recently diagnosed (<100 days, ages 6–45 years) T1D patients (NCT00505375). The primary outcome measure was insulin production (C-peptide at 2 years). Patients were assigned to either the abatacept (n = 77) or placebo (n = 35) arm. After 2 years, adjusted C-peptide AUC was 59% (95% CI 6.1–112) higher with abatacept (n = 73, 0.378 nmol/L) than with placebo (n = 30, 0.238 nmol/L; P = .0029). The difference between the groups continued throughout the trial, with an estimated 9.6 months delay (95% CI 3.47–15.6) in C-peptide reduction with abatacept. Infusion-related adverse events occurred more frequently with abatacept (22%) than with placebo (17%). There was no increase in infections or neutropenia on abatacept (42%, 9%) versus placebo (43%, 14%), respectively.[38] The safety profile of CTLA-4 may be preferable to other immunosuppressants in that it does that it does not deplete T cells.[39]

Treatment with abatacept slowed the rate of decline of β-cell function over a 2-year period, hinting that T-cell activation continues during the clinical diagnosis of T1D. However, the decrease in β-cell function still occurred despite continued dosing with abatacept. Although there was a 9.6 month delay, the rate of decline was parallel to that with placebo, suggesting that the effect of T-cell activation may diminish with time. Although this study marks progress, it remains to be seen whether the beneficial effect will continue after abatacept infusions cease.[38]

Antithymocyte Globulin

Antithymocyte globulin (ATG), a polyclonal anti–human-T-cell antibody, is used for conditioning before transplantation and cancer therapy due to its role in nonspecific T-cell depletion.[40] ATG has reversed T1D in NOD mice, but the results have not been reproducible in other animal models nor in clinical studies.[41] When T cells repopulate the immune system following ATG therapy, the balance between effector and regulatory T cells is shifted to favor regulatory T cells, giving this therapeutic approach a potential advantage in resetting the immune system in patients with autoimmune disorders.[42] ATG has been used alone or as combination therapy in various autoimmune conditions, including Wegener granulomatosis, lupus, rheumatoid arthritis, multiple sclerosis, scleroderma, aplastic anemia, and myelodysplastic syndrome, and T1D.[43–52] Although ATG does seem to have great promise in terms of efficacy, ATG is also associated with side effects such as cytokine release syndrome and serum sickness. Although concerning, these side effects may be mitigated in T1D patients by using lower doses of ATG than typically used in oncology. The NIH-funded Immune Tolerance Network is conducting a phase II evaluating ATG (thymoglobulin) in recently diagnosed T1D patients, with results expected in late 2013 (NCT00515099).

ATG and Granulocyte Colony-Stimulating Factor

ATG alone may be insufficient to provide long term benefit when used alone or may be associated with unacceptable side effects when used at an effective dose. The use of ATG in combination with another therapeutic agent may maximize efficacy (via synergy) and reduce risk associated with prolonged immunosuppression or side effects. One potential agent being studied in this regard is granulocyte colony-stimulating factor (GCSF). Notably, GCSF prevents T1D in NOD mice by inducing both tolerogenic dendritic cells and T-regulatory (Treg) cells. Additional preclinical data have shown that the combination of low-dose ATG and GCSF not only prevents, but also reverses diabetes in the NOD mouse.

Perhaps the most impressive support for this approach comes from a somewhat controversial clinical trial performed in Brazil. Investigators performed an aggressive and cutting-edge study in young T1D adults (14–31 years old) within 6 weeks of T1D diagnosis. Subjects were pretreated with cyclophosphamide and GCSF to mobilize the hematopoietic stem cells. Peripheral blood was collected by leukapheresis and cryopreserved. Subjects were then conditioned with cyclophosphamide and ATG before being reinfused with their previously harvested CD34+ cells.[53,54] This remarkable approach, referred to as autologous nonmyeloablative hematopoietic stem cell transplantation (AHST), nonselectively depletes immune cells and results in a long-term shift in the immune cell repertoire. (NCT00315133). Most impressively, 6 months after AHST, the mean total area under the C-peptide response curve was significantly higher than before treatment, and persisted at 24 months. After 6 months, anti-GAD antibody levels decreased and were stable at 24 months. Hemoglobin A1C was less than 7% in 13 of 14 patients. Twenty of 23 subjects were able to discontinue insulin, and 12 for a mean of 31 months. Adverse events included pneumonia in one subject and late endocrine dysfunction (hypothyroidism or hypogonadism) in two other subjects. There was no mortality.[53] As a result, small follow-up studies using this protocol are now being conducted in China and Poland.[55]

Despite the impressive results, many clinicians are reluctant to use such an aggressive therapy for a vulnerable T1D population. Therefore, the authors have attempted to deconstruct the Brazilian combination using the NOD mouse model to guide the development of a lower-risk therapy for humans. By excluding cyclophosphamide, and relying on a combination of only low-dose ATG and GCSF, we were recently able to demonstrate a durable reversal of diabetes in over 75% of NOD mice; while ATG alone was only able to reverse disease in 33% of animals.[56] In addition, we demonstrated that the combination therapy provided the most robust increase in regulatory T cells and, perhaps more importantly for clinical application, enabled reversal of diabetes at higher initial glucose values than ATG alone. Given these exciting preclinical data, our group established an analogous human trial designed to study the safety and potential efficacy of low-dose ATG (2.5 mg/kg total dose) and 12 weeks of pegylated GCSF therapy (Neulasta 6 mg every 2 weeks) (NCT01106157). This trial is expected to complete enrollment by the end of 2012 with initial first year data being reported at the end of 2013.

Cytokines

Cytokines have recently been targeted as an area for T1D interdiction. Cytokines affect T-cell responses (eg, interleukin [IL]-1, IL-2, IL-15, and IL-17) and participate in inflammation and β cell destruction. However, the role of cytokines in relation to autoimmune disorders remains poorly understood. One cytokine, IL-1, is selectively cytotoxic to rodent and in vitro human β cells. Several trials are evaluating various cytokine antagonists in newly diagnosed T1D, including anti-IL-1Ra (eg, anakinra, Kineret) (NCT00645840), a fully human anti-IL-1β antibody (canakinumab, Ilaris) (NCT00947427), and anti-IL-17 (secukinumab). Anakinra is used for patients with rheumatoid arthritis, and preclinical models suggest that it may also be useful for T1D patients (www.clinicaltrials.gov). It has recently completed a Phase II-III study in recent onset T1D subjects (NCT00711503). Although canakinumab was extremely safe, this therapeutic approach failed to demonstrate benefit in preservation of endogenous β-cell function when compared with placebo.[57] A similar trial using secukinumab (anti-IL-17 antibody) also reported a lack of benefit in new onset T1D patients.

One particular strategy involves the combined administration of rapamycin with agonistic IL-2-Fc and antagonistic IL-15-Fc fusion proteins. The concept is to limit effector T-cell activation and expansion (by blocking IL-15 signals) while promoting Treg cells (IL-2 and rapamycin). In the NOD mice, Proleukin promotes expansion of Treg cells, while sirolimus blocks expansion of effector T cells.[58] A Phase I trial evaluating Proleukin (IL-2) and sirolimus (rapamycin, Rapamune) in T1D subjects is ongoing with completion anticipated in September 2013 (NCT00525889). However, a pilot study was stopped due to worsening of C-peptide in treated subjects despite an increase in Treg cells. A Phase I/II clinical trial in T1D subjects (n = 25, within 2 years of diagnosis) with another anti IL-2 (aldesleukin) has just been completed, with results pending (NCT01353833).

Tumor necrosis factor α (TNF-α) is also a key mediator of the inflammatory response and has been implicated in autoimmune disorders, such as rheumatoid arthritis. In T1D, data from a phase II trial showed treatment with etanercept lowered HbA1c and increased endogenous insulin production.[59] However, subsequent studies have reported an increased incidence of T1D in patients being treated with etanercept for juvenile rheumatoid arthritis **Fig. 3**.[60,61]

Cell Therapies

The term "cell therapies" has evolved, expanding from the initial concept of using cells solely to provide a means of β-cell replacement (ie, islet transplantation and stem cell differentiation) to the more recent concepts of using cell therapies to provide immunoregulation. However, the two concepts are not exclusive of one another, clinical trials are currently investigating cell therapies aimed at using both potential capacities of cellular therapeutics. The ultimate "cure" for T1D individuals will likely involve a combination approach that uses cell therapy in some capacity to restore functional β-cell mass and reestablish tolerance to insulin and other β-cell antigens.

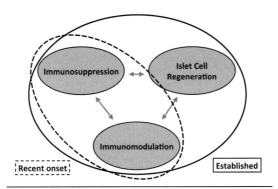

Fig. 3. Potential therapeutic targets. Three areas generally targeted for T1D intervention are immunosuppression (halting the autoimmune process), immunomodulation (altering the immunomodulatory response), and islet cell regeneration (replacing the destroyed β cells). In recent onset patients (<100 days), the desire is to halt the autoimmune process (immunosuppression) and to spare residual β cells (immunomodulation). However, in patients with long-standing diabetes, intervention in all three areas may be required. The goal of current therapeutics is to use combination therapies to target several pathways, with paramount consideration for safety.

β-cell replacement

Traditionally, β-cell replacement had referred to whole pancreas or islet transplant, but the shortage of donor pancreata has made this approach untenable. In addition, any success with β-cell replacement must be tempered by the sober reality of the primary alloimmune response, explaining why most islet grafts fail within the first 4 to 5 years, despite the use of potent immunosuppressants.[62] Therefore, novel approaches to augment or replace β cells have been explored, including stimulation of insulin secretion, islet neogenesis from progenitor cells, islet regeneration from existing β-cells, islet transplantation, and stem cell transplantation. We will focus on insulin secretion, islet transplantation, and stem cell since these are the areas with the most clinical data.

Islet transplantation—the Edmonton experience showed that about two-thirds of transplant recipients remained insulin-free posttransplant. Long-term data were disappointing, with fewer than 10% of patients remaining insulin-free by 5 years.[63] Based on the findings, the Edmonton protocol was modified with improvements to the islet purification techniques and changes to the immunosuppressant cocktail. A phase II trial assessing a steroid-free, calcineurin inhibitor-free immunosuppression protocol is currently underway (NCT00315627).

Stem cells may be manipulated to become insulin-producing cells by differentiating embryonic stem cells, pluripotent stem cells, or by the "reprogramming" of cells from their original phenotype (eg, pancreatic α cells, liver, spleen) into stem cells (induced pluripotent stem cells). Although stem cells like those described above have not yet been used in clinical trials to treat T1D, ongoing preclinical work has demonstrated the potential for these cell types to bridge the bench to bedside gap in subsequent years.

Autologous stem cells avoid alloimmune, but not autoimmune responses to the transplanted β-like cells. Encapsulation techniques using a protective permeable device to protect the fragile islets against the autoimmune response are currently being developed for commercial use. The capsule would ideally allow passage of glucose, but not autoimmune cells. Preliminary studies have been promising, but questions about the nutrient and insulin flow and capsule permeability to cytokines remain unanswered. Further clinical trials will determine the utility of such devices.

Cell-based immunomodulation

The concept behind cell-based immunomodulation is to compensate for the presumed lack of immunomodulatory (Treg cells) cells by either supplementing with additional Treg cells or inducing other cell types to transform into Treg cells. NOD models showed this could be done.[64,65] Hoping to expand on this, clinical studies performed similar experiments by isolating the patient's Treg cells, multiplying them outside the body, and reinfusing the cells into the subjects. Although conceptually simple, there are several logistical issues including identifying Treg cells (markers are not clearly defined) and finding them in the circulation (~5%–7% of CD4+ T cells).[66] Despite the challenges, cell therapies, including polyclonal regulatory T cells, antigen-specific regulatory T cells, and T cells modulated in vitro to produce anti-inflammatory cytokines in vivo[67] are being actively pursued. Currently, a novel Phase I study is evaluating the safety and feasibility of transfusing autologous CD4+CD127lo/-CD25+ polyclonal regulatory T cells (NCT01210664). Autologous Treg cells from T1D subjects are selected using specific T-cell markers (CD4, CD25, and CD127) and expanded through ex vivo methods. The Treg cells are then reinfused into the T1D subjects to inform future dose selection. Although the primary goal is assessing safety and feasibility, C-peptide measurement will be a secondary endpoint. Once hurdles with safety and feasibility are overcome, further trials will be initiated.

One source of stem cells that has been used in clinical trial is umbilical cord blood. Among several other potentially important cell types, umbilical cord blood contains a dense population of highly potent regulatory T cells. Because of its ease of collection, lack of ethical complications, and superb safety record, our group recently completed a phase I study investigating the potential for a single autologous cord blood infusion to induce immunoregulation through augmenting the frequency of regulatory T cells with hopes of preserving C-peptide in young children with T1D. Unfortunately, autologous cord blood infusion failed to demonstrate long-term preservation of C-peptide in our small open label study.[22] Further studies, including a small follow-up study using a randomized design with subjects receiving umbilical cord blood, vitamin D, and Docosahexaenoic acid (DHA) versus intensive therapy alone also failed to demonstrate benefit (NCT00873925, NCT00305344).[68]

In contrast to the safe but largely ineffective cell therapy approach explored using unmanipulated autologous cord blood infusion, the cell therapy approach used by Voltarelli and colleagues,[53] "nonmyeloablative hematopoietic stem cell transplant," was of extremely high risk but also considered by some to be the most effective therapy for new onset T1D studied to date. In addition, some have argued that the cell therapy provided by nonmyeloablative hematopoietic stem cell transplants is not a critical part of the therapy's efficacy and only serves to reduce the time during which patients are severely immunocompromised.

Mesenchymal stem cells (MSC) are thought, by most, to have little to no known allo-sensitivity. Theoretically, MSCs from any donor can be provided to any recipient, due to their ability to localize suppression of immune response in areas of inflammation. In vivo, MSCs have a limited life span, which may be favorable, given the perceived long-term concerns about immortalized stem cells. MSCs can also be re-dosed, due to their lack of inducing alloimmunity. Preclinical data from T1D animal models have shown the capacity of MSCs to promote β-cell repair, enhance insulin secretion, and facilitate islet allograft tolerance.[69,70] Remestemcel-L (Prochymal) is an intravenous formulation of MSCs, which are derived from the bone marrow of healthy adult donors and do not require that recipients be typed, matched or receive immunosuppression. An interim report of a phase II study using remestemcel-L in new-onset T1D patients showed that the therapy was well-tolerated, and that there were no differences in adverse events between the treatment and placebo groups. Of note, no patients experienced an infusion-related reaction despite the lack of matching or immunosuppression. Although there were no significant differences in stimulated C-peptide levels between the groups at 1 year, a trend toward fewer hypoglycemic events was seen for subjects treated with remestemcel-L as compared with controls. The patients will be followed for another year (total of two years), after which a final data analysis will be conducted (www.osiris.com) (NCT00690066).

Dendritic cells coordinate immune responses by presenting antigens on their cell surface in a form recognized by the immune system cells. Animal studies have confirmed that exogenous dendritic cells prevent autoimmunity and enables allograft survival.[71] Based on preliminary NOD studies confirming that altered dendritic cells can prevent T1D,[72] studies (NCT00445913) in established T1D patients (n = 10) have shown that treatment with nonmanipulated autologous dendritic cells or autologous dendritic cells directed ex vivo toward a costimulation-impaired immunologically suppressive state were safety tolerated. Of note, dendritic cells upregulated the frequency of a potentially beneficial B cells with a regulatory phenotype (B220+ CD11c- B-cells).[73] Future studies plan to target recent onset T1D patients.

As evidenced by several new potential targets and innovative therapeutic agents, the arena of cell-based therapies has expanded exponentially. We exercise cautious optimism knowing that each exciting discovery may only represent the tip of the iceberg **Table 1**.

Learning from the Past to Predict the Challenges of the Future

Since the 2010 edition of this text, several promising trials have demonstrated disappointing results. Yet learning from the negative trials is equally as important as celebrating the positive ones. For the industry-sponsored Phase 3 GAD65 (GAD-alum) (NCT00723411), 334 subjects (ages 10–20 years, fasting C-peptide >0.3 ng/mL, GAD65+, and <3 months of diagnosis) were treated with varying doses of GAD-alum or placebo. The primary outcome measure was stimulated C-peptide in the various groups between baseline and 15 months. Although the adverse events were infrequent and mild, the efficacy was disappointing: no difference in stimulated C-peptide between the study groups ($P = .10$), or in the secondary endpoints (HbA1c, daily insulin dose, hypoglycemia, maximum stimulated C-peptide).[13] Perhaps using GAD-alum in T1D prevention or starting it earlier in the disease process may be more effective. With this goal in mind, the Diabetes TrialNet GAD65-alum study group is evaluating GAD65-specific immune responses through tetramer assays, ELISPOT, flow markers, and transcript profiling.[74] Despite the negative results, these trials have illuminated our understanding of T1D epidemiology, pathogenesis, mechanism of action, and trial design and/or recruitment.

The current paradigm of preclinical testing in animal models, specifically the NOD mouse, remains imperfect. Critics of this model assert that therapies and "cures" in the inbred species have yet to demonstrate efficacy in humans.[75] In an elegant review, they conclude that timing, dose, and species-specific biology can critically impact therapeutic efficacy, and efforts to identify and minimize such issues may improve future translational efforts. Drug pharmacokinetic-pharmacodynamics, dosing ranges, and serum biomarkers need to be well-characterized to guide human dosing strategies. Lastly, unless, there are strong human data from pilot efforts or clinical data from other similarly mediated autoimmune diseases, potential T1D therapies should be tested in multiple animal models, with findings guiding future.

Similar to treatment strategies in oncology and other autoimmune disorders, T1D therapies may require synergistic approaches with combination agents to reverse autoimmunity, establish tolerance, and minimize side effects. Ideally, combination therapies should achieve three major goals: a safe therapeutic regimen that does not require long-term therapy, establishment of long-term tolerance, and regeneration of β-cell mass. T1D, unlike the other diseases, is not life-threatening, per se, and can be managed with daily insulin administration, with most individuals leading a productive life. Additionally, the disease generally afflicts a younger cohort. These factors give rise to logistical and regulatory challenges. Unless prior consent is given by the regulatory agencies, each agent within the combination needs extensive trials to receive approval. In addition, a study drug cannot be administered to younger children, until it has demonstrated safety and efficacy in the adult population. Significant adverse effects will prohibit agents from even being considered in young children. Safe, but ineffective therapies in adults may be aborted owing to commercial reasons, without further studies in children. T1D is a devastating, chronic disease, but, relative to other disorders, it is not common, making commercial drug development efforts less attractive. In efforts to entice drug development, the FDA has established the Orphan Drug Act,[76] which provides financial incentives to industry sponsors to encourage clinical trials in therapeutic areas affecting smaller populations (<200,000 United States

Table 1
T1D interdiction studies (partial listing)

Therapeutic Agent	NCT[a]
Published	
GAD-alum	NCT00723411 (EU)
	NCT00751842 (US)
Anti-CD3	NCT00378508, NCT00385697
Teplizumab	
Anti-CD3	NCT00451321, NCT00678886, NCT01123083
Otelixizumab	
Anti-CD20 rituximab	NCT00279305
Mycophenolate mofetil + anti-CD25	NCT00100178
CTLA-4	NCT00505375
Autologous nonmyeloablative	NCT00315133
transplantation	
Cord blood	NCT00305344
Anti-ILRa anakinra	NCT00645840
Completed enrollment	
Mesenchymal stem cells	NCT00690066
Cord blood phase 2 (+ vitamin d + omega 3	NCT00873925, NCT00305344
fatty acid)	
IL-2 plus sirolimus	NCT00525889
Enrolling	
INIT-II (intranasal insulin)	NCT00336674
Canakinumab	NCT00947427
ATG	NCT00515099
ATG + G-CSF	NCT01106157
Treg cells	NCT01210664
α-1-antitrypsin	NCT01183468, NCT01183455
DiaPep277	NCT01103284
Islet Transplantation	NCT00315627

This table represents a partial listing of past clinical trials and current ongoing trials in the effort to interdict T1D.

[a] Available at: www.clinicaltrials.gov. Accessed July 20, 2012.

patients). For example, a therapy specifically targeted for new onset type 1 diabetes patients could potentially qualify for orphan drug status. There are added financial incentives for developing therapeutic agents for pediatric patients (www.fda.gov).

Another challenge with T1D clinical trials is the lack of study endpoints. Although the outright reversal or prevention of T1D is an easily understood endpoint, measurements of incremental metabolic improvements, which guide us to that goal, are less easily agreed on. To compound this matter, is there are no imaging tools that directly visualize pancreatic function. Peak, basal, and area under the curve (AUC) C-peptide are commonly used metabolic endpoints but do not adequately reflect complex changes in islet function. Stimulated C-peptide is a well-accepted primary study endpoint, but it is only a surrogate measure of β-cell function. Secondary endpoints commonly comprise a composite of HbA1c, daily insulin use, and hypoglycemic events—again, acceptable but insufficient. Clinical trials have fortunately adopted the above study endpoints, so as to harmonize one aspect of this complex disease. Striving to find a clinically meaningful endpoint is critical for ensuring a successful "cure."

Assuming the ideal scenario of well-defined animal modes, a clear regulatory pathway, and solid study endpoints, there is the reality of finite monetary and human resources. The ability to use every agent with solid rationale in a timely manner is unfeasible. Factors, such as ease of delivery, agent cost, previous experience in other autoimmune disease, need for screening (in cases of T1D prevention), and applicability to large numbers of patients must all be considered in appropriately rank-ordering potential interventions.

Finally, if any or all of the above therapies were attainable and effective, the treatment would have to be acceptable to individuals with T1D. In pursuing the "cure," we must keep in mind, that application of even the most successful research interventions may not translate into similar clinical benefit for T1D patients who eagerly await "proven" interventions. Given the risks involved, patients may reasonably prefer multiple daily injections over stem cell therapy or even over a "successful" pancreas transplant.

SUMMARY

Accelerated by technological advances, we have recently witnessed an explosion of knowledge in understanding of T1D. Our grasp of the immune system has advanced significantly and allows us to target previously uncharted pathways. In parallel to the ongoing basic and clinical trials, advances in clinical care have dramatically improved the quality of life for T1D patients. Continuous glucose monitors and continuous subcutaneous insulin infusion devices will likely result in decreases in complication rates.

Reality dictates that a complete understanding of the underlying genetics and immunobiology of T1D is improbable. That said, our ever improving understanding of this complex disease process brings us closer to achieving our ultimate goals of prevention and cure. T1D is a burdensome disease with devastating consequences, so the need for a cure persists. Future prevention and intervention studies must be designed with an appreciation for the lessons learned from previous unsuccessful attempts. A multipronged approach (eg, agents targeting immunosuppression, immunomodulation, and islet regeneration) has the highest probability of success. Most importantly, global collaborations among those in academia, clinical practice, industry, government regulators, advocacy groups, and individuals with T1D are mandatory in our urgent quest for a cure.

REFERENCES

1. Skyler J. Approaches to interdicting type 1 diabetes. International Diabetes Monitor 2010;22(3):132–37.
2. Haller MJ, Atkinson MA, Schatz DA. Efforts to prevent and halt autoimmune beta cell destruction. Endocrinol Metab Clin North Am 2010;39(3):527–39.
3. Gallagher MP, Goland RS, Greenbaum CJ. Making progress: preserving beta cells in type 1 diabetes. Ann N Y Acad Sci 2011;1243:119–34.
4. Atkinson MA, Maclaren NK, Luchetta R. Insulitis and diabetes in NOD mice reduced by prophylactic insulin therapy. Diabetes 1990;39(8):933–7.
5. Diabetes Prevention Trial–Type 1 Diabetes Study Group. Effects of insulin in relatives of patients with type 1 diabetes mellitus. N Engl J Med 2002;346:1685–91.

6. Vehik K, Cuthbertson D, Ruhlig H, et al. DPT-1 and TrialNet Study Groups. Long-term outcome of individuals treated with oral insulin: diabetes prevention trial-type 1 (DPT-1) oral insulin trial. Diabetes Care 2011;34(7):1585–90.

7. Harrison LC, Honeyman MC, Steele CE, et al. Pancreatic beta-cell function and immune responses to insulin after administration of intranasal insulin to humans at risk for type 1 diabetes. Diabetes Care 2004;27(10):2348–55.

8. Fourlanos S, Perry C, Gellert SA, et al. Evidence that nasal insulin induces immune tolerance to insulin in adults with autoimmune diabetes. Diabetes 2011;60:1237–45.

9. INIT II Study Web Site. 2010. Available at: http://www.diabetestrials.org/initii.html. Accessed July 18, 2012.

10. Orban T, Farkas K, Jalahej H, et al. Autoantigen-specific regulatory T cells induced in patients with type 1 diabetes mellitus by insulin B-chain immuno-therapy. J Autoimmun 2010;34(4):408–15.

11. Tisch R, Yang XD, Liblau RS, et al. Administering glutamic acid decarboxylase to NOD mice prevents diabetes. J Autoimmun 1994;7(6):845–50.

12. Ludvigsson J, Faresjo M, Hjorth M, et al. GAD treatment and insulin secretion in recent-onset type 1 diabetes. N Engl J Med 2008;359(18):1909–20.

13. Ludvigsson J, Krisky D, Casas R, et al. GAD65 antigen therapy in recently diag-nosed type 1 diabetes mellitus. N Engl J Med 2012;366(5):433–42.

14. Silverstein J, Maclaren N, Riley W, et al. Immunosuppression with azathioprine and prednisone in recent-onset insulin-dependent diabetes mellitus. N Engl J Med 1988;319(10):599–604.

15. Bougneres PF, Carel JC, Castano L, et al. Cyclosporin and childhood diabetes: preliminary findings of the Saint Vincent de Paul trial. Journ Annu Diabetol Hotel Dieu 1987;181–6 [in French].

16. Carel JC, Boitard C, Eisenbarth G, et al. Cyclosporine delays but does not prevent clinical onset in glucose intolerant pre-type 1 diabetic children. J Autoimmun 1996;9(6):739–45.

17. Eisenbarth GS, Srikanta S, Jackson R, et al. Anti-thymocyte globulin and predni-sone immunotherapy of recent onset type 1 diabetes mellitus. Diabetes Res 1985;2(6):271–6.

18. Gale EA. European Nicotinamide Diabetes Intervention Trial (ENDIT): a rando-mised controlled trial of intervention before the onset of type 1 diabetes. Lancet 2004;363(9413):925–31.

19. Bohmer KP, Kolb H, Kuglin B, et al. Linear loss of insulin secretory capacity during the last six months preceding IDDM. No effect of antiedematous therapy with ketotifen. Diabetes Care 1994;17(2):138–41.

20. Huppmann M, Baumgarten A, Ziegler AG, et al. Neonatal Bacille Calmette-Guerin vaccination and type 1 diabetes. Diabetes Care 2005;28(5):1204–6.

21. Haller MJ, Wasserfall CH, McGrail KM, et al. Autologous umbilical cord blood transfusion in very young children with type 1 diabetes. Diabetes Care 2009; 32(11):2041–6.

22. Zhang B, Lu Y, Campbell-Thompson M, et al. Alpha1-antitrypsin protects beta-cells from apoptosis. Diabetes 2007;56(5):1316–23.

23. Huurman VA, van der Meide PE, Duinkerken G, et al. Immunological efficacy of heat shock protein 60 peptide DiaPep277 therapy in clinical type I diabetes. Clin Exp Immunol 2008;152(3):488–97.

24. Study design of the Trial to Reduce IDDM in the Genetically at Risk (TRIGR). Pediatr Diabetes 2007;8(3):117–37.

25. Raz I, Elias D, Avron A, et al. Beta-cell function in new-onset type 1 diabetes and immunomodulation with a heat-shock protein peptide (DiaPep277): a randomised, double-blind, phase II trial. Lancet 2001;358(9295):1749–53.

26. Herold KC, Bluestone JA, Montag AG, et al. Prevention of autoimmune diabetes with nonactivating anti-CD3 monoclonal antibody. Diabetes 1992;41(3):385–91.

27. Sherry NA, Chen W, Kushner JA, et al. Exendin-4 improves reversal of diabetes in NOD mice treated with anti-CD3 monoclonal antibody by enhancing recovery of beta-cells. Endocrinology 2007;148(11):5136–44.

28. Keymeulen B, Vandemeulebroucke E, Ziegler AG, et al. Insulin needs after CD3-antibody therapy in new-onset type 1 diabetes. N Engl J Med 2005;352(25):2598–608.

29. Haller MJ, Schatz DA. CD3-antibody therapy in new-onset type 1 diabetes mellitus. N Engl J Med 2005;353(19):2086–7.

30. Sherry N, Hagopian W, Ludvigsson J, et al, Protégé Trial Investigators. Teplizumab for treatment of type 1 diabetes (Protégé study): 1-year results from a randomised, placebo-controlled trial. Lancet 2011;378(9790):487–97.

31. Available at: http://us.gsk.com/html/medianews/pressreleases/2011/2011_press release_10039.htm. Accessed July 18, 2012.

32. Pescovitz MD, Greenbaum CJ, Krause-Steinrauf H, et al, Type 1 Diabetes TrialNet Anti-CD20 Study Group. Rituximab, B-lymphocyte depletion, and preservation of beta-cell function. N Engl J Med 2009;361:2143–52.

33. Xiu Y, Wong CP, Bouaziz JD, et al. B lymphocyte depletion by CD20 monoclonal antibody prevents diabetes in nonobese diabetic mice despite isotype-specific differences in Fc gamma R effector functions. J Immunol 2008; 180(5):2863–75.

34. Fiorina P, Vergani A, Dada S, et al. Targeting CD22 reprograms B-cells and reverses autoimmune diabetes. Diabetes 2008;57(11):3013–24.

35. Gottlieb PA, Quinlan S, Krause-Steinrauf H, et al. Failure to preserve beta-cell function with mycophenolate mofetil and daclizumab combined therapy in patients with new onset type 1 diabetes. Diabetes Care 2010;33(4):826–32.

36. Rudd CE, Taylor A, Schneider H. CD28 and CTLA-4 coreceptor expression and signal transduction. Immunol Rev 2009;229(1):12–26.

37. Korolija M, Renar IP, Hadzija M, et al. Association of PTPN22 C1858T and CTLA-4 A49G polymorphisms with Type 1 Diabetes in Croatians. Diabetes Res Clin Pract 2009;86(3):e54–7.

38. Orban T, Bundy B, Becker DJ, et al, Type 1 Diabetes TrialNet Abatacept Study Group. Co-stimulation modulation with abatacept in patients with recent-onset type 1 diabetes: a randomised, double-blind, placebo-controlled trial. Lancet 2011;378(9789):412–9.

39. Van Belle TL, Coppieters KT, von Herrath MG. Type 1 diabetes: etiology, immunology, and therapeutic strategies. Physiol Rev 2011;91:79–118.

40. Mohty M. Mechanisms of action of antithymocyte globulin: T-cell depletion and beyond. Leukemia 2007;21(7):1387–94.

41. Bresson D, von Herrath MG. Anti-thymoglobulin (ATG) treatment does not reverse type 1 diabetes in the acute virally induced rat insulin promoter-lymphocytic choriomeningitis virus (RIP-LCMV) model. Clin Exp Immunol 2011;163(3):375–80.

42. Saccardi R, Kozak T, Bocelli-Tyndall C, et al. Autologous stem cell transplantation for progressive multiple sclerosis: update of the European Group for Blood and Marrow Transplantation autoimmune diseases working party database. Mult Scler 2006;12(6):814–23.

43. Fassas A, Anagnostopoulos A, Kazis A, et al. Peripheral blood stem cell transplantation in the treatment of progressive multiple sclerosis: first results of a pilot study. Bone Marrow Transplant 1997;20(8):631–8.
44. Frickhofen N, Heimpel H, Kaltwasser JP, et al. Antithymocyte globulin with or without cyclosporin A: 11-year follow-up of a randomized trial comparing treatments of aplastic anemia. Blood 2003;101(4):1236–42.
45. Kool J, de Keizer RJ, Siegert CE. Antithymocyte globulin treatment of orbital Wegener granulomatosis: a follow-up study. Am J Ophthalmol 1999;127(6):738–9.
46. McSweeney PA, Nash RA, Sullivan KM, et al. High-dose immunosuppressive therapy for severe systemic sclerosis: initial outcomes. Blood 2002;100(5): 1602–10.
47. Molldrem JJ, Leifer E, Bahceci E, et al. Antithymocyte globulin for treatment of the bone marrow failure associated with myelodysplastic syndromes. Ann Intern Med 2002;137(3):156–63.
48. Musso M, Porretto F, Crescimanno A, et al. Intense immunosuppressive therapy followed by autologous peripheral blood selected progenitor cell reinfusion for severe autoimmune disease. Am J Hematol 2001;66(2):75–9.
49. Rosenfeld S, Follmann D, Nunez O, et al. Antithymocyte globulin and cyclosporine for severe aplastic anemia: association between hematologic response and long-term outcome. JAMA 2003;289(9):1130–5.
50. Stratton RJ, Wilson H, Black CM. Pilot study of anti-thymocyte globulin plus mycophenolate mofetil in recent-onset diffuse scleroderma. Rheumatology (Oxford) 2001;40(1):84–8.
51. Schatz DA, Riley WJ, Silverstein JH, et al. Long-term immunoregulatory effects of therapy with corticosteroids and anti-thymocyte globulin. Immunopharmacol Immunotoxicol 1989;11(2–3):269–87.
52. Saudek F, Havrdova T, Boucek P, et al. Polyclonal anti-T-cell therapy for type 1 diabetes mellitus of recent onset. Rev Diabet Stud 2004;1(2):80–8.
53. Voltarelli JC, Couri CE, Stracieri AB, et al. Autologous nonmyeloablative hematopoietic stem cell transplantation in newly diagnosed type 1 diabetes mellitus. JAMA 2007;297(14):1568–76.
54. Couri CE, Oliveira MC, Stracieri AB, et al. C-peptide levels and insulin independence following autologous nonmyeloablative hematopoietic stem cell transplantation in newly diagnosed type 1 diabetes mellitus. JAMA 2009;301(15): 1573–9.
55. Gu W, Hu J, Wang W, Li L, et al. Diabetic Ketoacidosis at Diagnosis Influences Complete Remission After Treatment with Hematopoietic Stem Cell Transplantation in Adolescents with Type 1 Diabetes. Diabetes Care 2012;35:1413–9.
56. Parker MJ, Xue S, Alexander JJ, et al. Immune depletion with cellular mobilization imparts immunoregulation and reverses autoimmune diabetes in nonobese diabetic mice. Diabetes 2009;58(10):2277–84.
57. Moran A. Canakinumab, and anti-IL-1 Monoclonal Antibody in Recent-Onset Type 1 Diabetes. 72nd Scientific Sessions, American Diabetes Association. Philadelphia, June 8-12, 2012.
58. Rabinovitch A, Suarez-Pinzon WL, Shapiro AM, et al. Combination therapy with sirolimus and interleukin-2 prevents spontaneous and recurrent autoimmune diabetes in NOD mice. Diabetes 2002;51:638–45.
59. Mastrandrea L, Yu JH, Behrens T, et al. Etanercept treatment in children with new-onset type 1 diabetes: pilot randomized, placebo-controlled, double-blind study. Diabetes Care 2009;32(7):1244–9.

60. Boulton JG, Bourne JT. Unstable diabetes in a patient receiving anti-TNF-α for rheumatoid arthritis. Rheumatology 2007;46(1):178–9.
61. Tack CJ, Kleijwegt FS, Van Riel PL, et al. Development of type 1 diabetes in a patient treated with anti-TNF-α therapy for active rheumatoid arthritis. Diabetologia 2009;52(7):1442–4.
62. Harlan DM, Kenyon NS, Korsgren O, et al, Immunologyof Diabetes Study. Current advances and travails in islet transplantation. Diabetes 2009;58:2175–84.
63. Ryan EA, Paty BW, Senior PA, et al. Five-year follow-up after clinical islet transplantation. Diabetes 2005;54:2060–9.
64. Tang Q, Henriksen KJ, Bi M, et al. In vitro- expanded antigen-specific regulatory T cells suppress autoimmune diabetes. J Exp Med 2004;199:1455–65.
65. Tarbell KV, Yamazaki S, Olson K, et al. CD25+ CD4+T cells, expanded with dendritic cells presenting a single autoantigenic peptide, suppress autoimmune diabetes. J Exp Med 2004;199:1467–77.
66. Baecher-Allan C, Brown JA, Freeman GJ, et al. CD4+CD25 high regulatory cells in human peripheral blood. J Immunol 2001;167:1245–53.
67. Tang Q, Bluestone JA. The Foxp3+ regulatory T cell: a jack of all trades, master of regulation. Nat Immunol 2008;9(3):239–44.
68. Haller MJ, Wasserfall C, McGrail K, et al. Pilot Study of Autologous Umbilical Cord Blood (UCB) Transfusion Followed by Docosahexanoic Acid (DHA) and Vitamin D (VitD) Supplementation in Children with Type 1 Diabetes (T1D). Philadelphia: American Diabetes Association, Scientific Sessions; June 8-12, 2012.
69. Fiorina P, Jurewicz M, Augello A, et al. Immunomodulatory function of bone marrow-derived mesenchymal stem cells in experimental autoimmune type 1 diabetes. J Immunol 2009;183(2):993–1004.
70. Madec AM, Mallone R, Afonso G, et al. Mesenchymal stem cells protect NOD mice from diabetes by inducing regulatory T cells. Diabetologia 2009;52(7): 1391–9.
71. McCurry KR, Colvin BL, Zahorchak AF, et al. Regulatory dendritic cell therapy in organ transplantation. Transpl Int 2006;19:525–38.
72. Ma L, Qian S, Liang X, et al. Prevention of diabetes in NOD mice by administration of dendritic cells deficient in nuclear transcription factor-kappaB activity. Diabetes 2003;52(8):1976–85.
73. Giannoukakis N, Phillips B, Finegold D. Phase I (safety) study of autologous tolerogenic dendritic cells in type 1 diabetic patients. Diabetes Care 2011;34(9): 2026–32.
74. Greenbaum CJ, Schatz DA, Haller MJ, et al. Through the fog: recent clinical trials to preserve β-cell function in type 1 diabetes. Diabetes 2012;61(6):1323–30.
75. Shoda LK, Young DL, Ramanujan S, et al. A comprehensive review of interventions in the NOD mouse and implications for translation. Immunity 2005;23(2): 115–26 [PubMed: 16111631].
76. Available at: http://www.fda.gov/ForIndustry/DevelopingProductsforRareDiseases Conditions/HowtoapplyforOrphanProductDesignation/ucm135125. Accessed August 31, 2012.

Update on Turner and Noonan Syndromes

Elizabeth Chacko, MD[a], Evan Graber, DO[a],
Molly O. Regelmann, MD[a], Elizabeth Wallach, MD[a],
Gertrude Costin, MD[a,b], Robert Rapaport, MD[a,*]

KEYWORDS

- Turner syndrome • Noonan syndrome • Growth
- Recombinant human growth hormone • Estrogen therapy

KEY POINTS

- Turner and Noonan syndromes have short stature as a common feature. Both conditions present clinicians with a challenging array of genetic, developmental, cardiovascular, and psychosocial issues.
- Recombinant human growth hormone (hGH) has been approved by the Food and Drug Administration for treatment of short stature in both conditions.
- Long-term follow-up in patients with Turner syndrome treated with hGH have clearly indicated a beneficial effect on adult stature. Although it seems that treatment can be safely initiated in early childhood, the exact age of start of treatment remains controversial.
- Although treatment with hGH in children with Noonan syndrome has shown to increase short-term height velocity comparable to that noted in Turner syndrome, its effect on adult height has yet to be proven.
- Both syndromes, although sharing some common clinical features, have specific characteristic screening, treatment, management, and follow-up pathways.

INTRODUCTION

Turner syndrome (TS) and Noonan syndrome (NS) have short stature as a constant feature; however, both conditions can present clinicians with a challenging array of genetic, cardiovascular, developmental, and psychosocial issues. In recent years, important advances have been achieved in each of these areas. This article reviews these two syndromes and provides updates on recent developments in diagnostic evaluation, growth and development, psychological issues, and treatment options

---

Disclosure: No conflicts of interest to declare.
[a] Division of Pediatric Endocrinology and Diabetes, Mount Sinai School of Medicine, 1 Gustave L. Levy Place Box 1616, New York, NY 10029, USA; [b] Keck Medical School, University Southern California, 1975 Zonal Avenue, Los Angeles, CA 90089, USA
* Corresponding author.
E-mail address: Robert.rapaport@mountsinai.org

Endocrinol Metab Clin N Am 41 (2012) 713–734
http://dx.doi.org/10.1016/j.ecl.2012.08.007
0889-8529/12/$ – see front matter © 2012 Elsevier Inc. All rights reserved.

for children with TS and NS. Treatment with recombinant human growth hormone (hGH) for improving adult height was approved by the Food and Drug Administration (FDA) for both conditions. Long-term studies in TS patients have indicated that early appropriate use of hGH increased their adult height.[1,2] The combination of hGH and low-dose estrogen suggested an added benefit on growth and adult height, as well as on potential neurocognitive and behavioral benefits.[3] In patients with NS, treatment with hGH has resulted in short-term increases in growth velocity and modest improvement in adult height; however, their follow-up has been shorter than in those with TS.[4–7] Further prospective studies are needed to confirm the long-term effects of hGH on adult height in patients with NS.

TS

TS results from a partial or complete absence (monosomy) of one X chromosome or the presence of a structurally abnormal X chromosome.[8] Although approximately 50% of affected individuals have 45, X karyotype and 20% to 30% have mosaicism (45, X, and at least one other cell line), the rest have various structural abnormalities (deletions of short and long arm of X chromosome, duplications, ring chromosomes).[9] TS affects 1 per 1500 to 1 per 2500 live female births.[8,10] The disorder causes short stature, skeletal anomalies, complete or partial lack of sexual development, and infertility; as well as cardiac, endocrine, and kidney abnormalities, and a propensity for autoimmune disease.

Prenatal Diagnosis

Sex chromosome abnormalities are increasingly being detected prenatally by chorionic villous sampling or amniocentesis. Sonography is a useful tool in the prenatal diagnosis of TS. The most common sonographic findings include nuchal cystic hygroma, nonimmune hydrops, and increased nuchal translucency.[11] Other ultrasound findings suggestive of TS include coarctation of the aorta, left-sided cardiac defects, renal anomalies, oligohydramnios, polyhydramnios, and intrauterine growth retardation. Diagnosis of TS can also be suspected in abnormal triple or quadruple maternal serum screening (α-fetoprotein, human chorionic gonadotropin, inhibin A, and unconjugated estriol).[12] However, neither ultrasound nor maternal serum screening are 100% diagnostic and confirmation by karyotype (via amniocentesis or chorionic villus sampling) is necessary.[12,13] The occurrence of 45, X karyotype is about 1% to 2% in all female conceptions leading to a 90% or greater fetal loss.[14,15]

Early detection can help identify cardiac malformations such as bicuspid aortic valve that require treatment to prevent complications. Early diagnosis helps prevent or remediate growth failure, hearing problems, and learning difficulties. Although the recurrence risk for TS is not increased, genetic counseling is recommended for families who have had a pregnancy or child with TS. Prenatal counseling should involve the discussion of the variable features of TS, the likelihood of congenital heat disease, kidney abnormalities, short stature, ovarian failure, and their management. It should be emphasized that most individuals with TS have normal intelligence, but may have specific learning disabilities.[12]

Postnatal Diagnosis

Diagnosis of TS requires a peripheral blood karyotype. If there is a strong clinical suspicion despite a normal peripheral blood karyotype, a second tissue (eg, skin) should be examined. Individuals with the 45, X karyotype tend to have a more characteristic phenotype than those who are mosaic with a normal cell line (45, X/46 XX or 45,

X/46 XY). Testing for the Y chromosome should be performed in all patients (or fetuses) with TS because the Y chromosome confers an increased risk for gonado-blastoma and subsequent transformation to a germ cell tumor. Gonadoblastoma was reported in 33% of children with TS with Y-positive material.[16,17] Testing for the Y chromosome can be achieved with DNA or fluorescent in situ hybridization (FISH) studies using a Y centromere probe, supplemented by long and short arm probes.[12] Some patients with TS have a dicentric Y chromosome (45, X/46, X, dic Y), while in others the Y chromosome may be represented by only a fragment (45, X/46, XY +fra) and Y-specific probes can be used to establish its origin. In patients with TS, SRY gene mutations have also been described and have been implicated in the develop-ment of gonadal lesions.[18] It is important to inform parents regarding the finding of the Y chromosome material and regarding gender identity issues in a manner that minimizes psychological harm. Laparoscopic gonadectomy is recommended for patients who have a Y cell line. Because some women with TS and the Y chromosome mosaicism may undergo spontaneous puberty and occasionally become pregnant, follicle or oocyte preservation should be discussed before gonadectomy.[9,12]

Indications for Karyotype

The diagnosis of TS should be considered in all girls with unexplained short stature or pubertal delay and short women with lack of complete sexual development and/or inability to conceive. It should also be considered in any female with edema of the hands or feet, nuchal folds, left-sided cardiac defects, low posterior hairline, low-set ears, cubitus valgus, short fourth metacarpal, triangular facies, high-arched palate, multiple pigmented nevi, nail hypoplasia, hyperconvex uplifted nail, chronic otitis media, or markedly elevated follicle-stimulating hormone (FSH) levels.

Medical Care in TS

In 2007, the international consensus guidelines regarding the care of girls and women with TS were published.[12] The extent to which these recommendations have resulted in changes in the medical care of young girls and adolescents with TS is unknown. A study in 2009, of more than 500 adults with TS reported that only 3.5% underwent the medical follow-up that was recommended in the guidelines.[12,19]

Of 128 girls with TS, mean age 13.2 ± 0.5 years, recommended surveillance was followed in only 50% of the patients.[20] Given the high rates of related morbidities, it is important to place emphasis on routine screening for cardiac defects, thyroid, celiac, and liver diseases. Although some changes in medical practice have been made, there is still a need to emphasize the importance of continued education of all primary and subspecialty care physicians, involved in the care of these individuals.

Cardiovascular System

Congenital cardiovascular disease affects approximately half of individuals with TS and is the major cause of mortality in adults.[21] Bicuspid aortic valve is the most common congenital cardiac malformation, whereas coarctation of aorta accounts for approximately 10% of cardiac abnormalities in women with TS.[22] A major concern in patients with TS is the occurrence of aortic dilatation, dissection, or rupture. Systemic hypertension is an important treatable risk factor for aortic enlargement and dissection.[23,24] Hypertension is estimated to occur in 25% of adolescents and 50% of adults with TS.[15] Some of the attributable causes of hypertension reported in TS include renal disease and aortic coarctation.[22]

Cardiovascular screening should include blood pressure monitoring, echocardio-gram (ECHO) and cardiovascular MRI. All newly diagnosed individuals with TS should have a baseline cardiology evaluation and a two-dimensional and color Doppler ECHO. If ECHO is inadequate, CT scan or cardiac MRI should be considered. In addition to anatomic screening, newly diagnosed TS patients should have a baseline ECG and routine evaluation of blood pressure.[20]

All left-sided cardiac anomalies seen in TS may increase the risk of infectious endocarditis. Therefore, it is important that patients receive prophylactic antibiotics before dental or surgical procedures.[22] TS patients with cardiac anomalies require long-term cardiology follow-up. For patients without identified cardiovascular defects, routine pediatric care with continued monitoring of blood pressure is recommended. Cardiovascular reassessment should be done at the time of pediatric transition to adult care. For TS adults who are normotensive and without any underlying cardiovascular disease, it is important to reevaluate aortic dimensions at 5 to10 year intervals.[12]

Hypertensive patients should have aortic dimensions determined on a regular basis. TS patients with multiple risk factors (bicuspid aortic valve, dilated aortic root, and hypertension) need to be counseled about pregnancy and appropriate exercise programs that do not stress the heart.[12] Preconception assessment should include cardiology evaluation with MRI of the aorta. Relative contraindications to pregnancy in TS women include bicuspid aortic valve, previous surgically repaired cardiovascular defect, or current evidence of systemic hypertension or aortic dilatation.[12] Close cardiology monitoring over the course of the pregnancy and during the postpartum period is mandatory.

Skeletal System

Short stature is a common clinical feature of TS. The growth pattern is characterized by intrauterine growth retardation, growth failure during early childhood (as early as 1 year), absent pubertal growth spurt, and mild skeletal dysplasias.[10,12,17] Skeletal abnormalities include an increased risk for hip dislocation in infancy and a higher risk for scoliosis and kyphosis. Other clinical findings may include short neck, cubitus valgus, genu valgum, and short fourth metacarpals. Madelung deformity, although infrequent, has been reported.

Individuals with TS are typically not growth hormone (GH) deficient, but seem to have an impaired response to endogenous GH, leading to diminished growth velocity. A disruption in the GH and insulin-like growth factor (IGF) axis is thought to play a role in the growth failure seen in individuals with TS. Increased IGFBP3 proteolytic activity combined with low levels of circulating free IGF-I and increased IGF-II have been found in individuals with TS.[25] Haploinsufficiency of the short-stature homeobox-containing gene (SHOX), which is located on the distal end at Xp22.3 and Yp11.3 in the pseudoautosomal region, is thought to be partly responsible for short stature in TS.

GH Treatment in TS

The primary goal of hGH therapy in TS is to normalize height as early in childhood as possible, so that the patient can maintain a normal stature through development and reach a good adult height. Untreated individuals with TS achieve an average adult stature of 20 cm shorter than that of their peers.[9] Treatment with hGH for patients with TS was approved by the FDA in 1996 and has since been the standard of care. Multiple publications, including clinical trials[26–28] and observational studies,[29–31] have demonstrated the beneficial effect of hGH on adult stature and its increased efficacy when treatment was initiated in early childhood.[1,2] The factors predictive of a better height outcome include taller mean parental height, relatively tall height and young age at treatment initiation, long duration of therapy, and a higher dose of hGH.[32–37] There is variability in the effect of hGH and much attention is currently focused on identifying the genetic factors underlying this variation. The influence of the parental origin of the X-chromosome on adult height after hGH therapy was evaluated in a controlled study.[38] The results indicated that individuals with a maternal X-chromosome grew more than those with a paternal X-chromosome by a mean of 3.37 cm (95% CI, 0.66–6.09) and this X-linked imprinting effect explained 36% of the total height gain with hGH.[38] A more recent study of 180 patients with 45, X karyotype, reported that the parental origin of the X-chromosome had no influence on growth before or during hGH treatment or on adult stature. These results raise questions about the role of the imprinted genes involved in growth and located on the X-chromosome.[39] Additional studies are needed to confirm the effect of the parental origin of the X-chromosome on other characteristics of TS.

Clinical studies regarding hGH therapy in TS have reported variable results, with most showing positive height gains ranging from increases of 5 to 8 cm to as much as 15 to 17 cm.[40,41] The variability has been attributed to different GH treatment protocols and different methodologies.[41,42]

The optimal age of hGH therapy initiation is still debated. In the past decade, improved guidance in diagnosing TS have led to earlier recognition of TS, thereby allowing for earlier start of treatment. A multicenter clinical trial reported that treatment with hGH in children with TS, initiated between 9 months and 4 years of age (mean age 2.0 years), restored height to within the normal range in approximately 93% of the girls before reaching the age of 6 years.[1] Results from an open-label, multicenter phase III study in which 61 girls with TS, younger than 4 years old, treated with hGH (0.245–0.35 mg/kg/wk) for 4 years, indicated that by age 6.6 years, 80% achieved a height greater than 1.09 SD than that of the untreated girls.[2] Based on reports from various studies, the Turner Syndrome Study Consensus Group[12] suggested starting hGH therapy as soon as growth failure is demonstrated. However, initiation of hGH therapy in TS is usually delayed, with a mean age at initiation of 8.6 ± 4.0 years.[42] Continuation of GH therapy for greater than or equal to 3 years resulted in 62.5% of patients achieving a height standard deviation score within the normal population range.[42] The National Cooperative Growth Study reported that the mean age of hGH therapy initiation was 9.0 ± 3.8 years.[43] Although, the general consensus is that hGH can be safely initiated at younger ages than originally recommended, how young the age should be, remains undetermined. More recent data emphasize the clinical importance of early diagnosis and early initiation of hGH therapy and its continuation throughout the growth period to optimize height gains in individuals with TS. **Table 1** summarizes selected published results on adult height gains in individuals with TS treated with hGH.[1,2,27,42,44]

Although treatment with hGH in young girls with TS has an overall favorable safety profile, hGH therapy-related adverse effects should be monitored. It is recommended that IGF-I, glucose, and insulin levels, be routinely monitored and maintained within normal range during hGH therapy.[2] Likewise, occurrences of coarse facial features and/or enlargement of hands and feet should also be monitored. The incidence of specific adverse side effects, including intracranial hypertension, scoliosis, pancreatitis, and slipped capital femoral epiphysis, were higher in patients with TS receiving hGH compared with matched patients receiving hGH for other indications.[45] There is a need for long-term follow-up regarding the safety of hGH treatment, especially in those who start hGH at a very young age and continue treatment for a longer duration.

Ovarian Failure and Pubertal Induction

Ovarian failure is a common manifestation of girls with TS. Individuals with 45, X karyotype usually have prenatal degeneration of ovarian follicles that lead to streak gonads

Table 1
Studies on GH therapy and adult height gain in TS

Study	hGH-Treated Patients (n)	Mean Age of Start (Y) (Mean ± SD)	Height SDS at Baseline (Mean ± SD)	Initial hGH Dose (mg/kg/wk)	Mean Treatment Duration (Y) (Mean ± SD/Mean)	Height SDS Gain (From Baseline to Adult Height)
Davenport et al,[1] 2007	45	1.98 ± 1.01	−1.42 ± 1.0	0.35	2.0	1.1 ± 0.6
Linglart et al,[2] 2011	43[b]	2.6 ± 0.6	−2.6 ± 0.6	0.245	4	0.98[d]
	18[c]	2.6 ± 1.3	−1.6 ± 0.4	0.35	4	0.98[d]
Stephure et al,[a,27] 2005	61	10.3 ± 1.8	−0.2 ± 0.9[e]	0.30[f]	5.7 ± 1.6	1.6 ± 0.6[e]
Ross et al,[42] 2011	382	8.62 ± 4.03	−2.58 ± 0.9	0.357[g]	4.54	(0.43, 0.89, 0.92)[h]
Blum et al,[44] 2009	158	10.9 ± 3.1	−2.9 ± 0.8	0.31 ± 0.09	5.6 ± 2.3	1.2 ± 0.8

Abbreviation: SDS, standard deviation score.
[a] The Canadian Growth Hormone Advisory Committee.
[b] Standard-dose group (0.035 mg/kg/d).
[c] Low-dose group (0.05 mg/kg/d).
[d] Height SDS at start of GH treatment −2.33 ± 0.73 and height SDS at end of study −1.35 ± 0.86.
[e] Age-specific TS.
[f] GH dose was given 6 days per week.
[g] GH dose 0.051 ± 0.0098.
[h] Duration of hGH therapy: 1 y, <3 y, and ≥3 y, respectively.

and absent pubertal development.[46,47] More than 90% of affected girls with TS require hormone replacement therapy (HRT) for pubertal initiation and completion of growth.[48,49] Although 20% to 30% of girls with TS have spontaneous pubertal development, only a few continue to maintain ovarian function.[12,50] Spontaneous menarche can occur in individuals with mosaicism for 46 XX and terminal Xp deletions. Poor potential for fertility is associated with Xq deletions, 45 XO, ring X chromosome, and mosaicism including 46 XY.[51] Spontaneous pregnancies are rare (2%–5%) and are usually associated with mosaic karyotype or distal Xp deletions.[15,51,52]

Markers of ovarian reserve include serum gonadotropins, antral follicle counts, inhibin A and B, and antimüllerian hormone (AMH). Elevated gonadotropins and hypoplastic uterus or ovaries indicate poor potential for fertility. Serum levels of AMH and inhibin A can be used as screening tests for assessing ovarian reserve.[51] Undetectable inhibin B levels in childhood are predictive of ovarian failure and lack of spontaneous puberty.[46,51]

Women with TS are generally infertile, although a few do achieve spontaneous pregnancy. Fertility expectations have changed in the last 3 decades for individuals with TS. Various assisted reproductive techniques are available for achieving pregnancy. Women with TS who have functional ovaries should receive counseling regarding the timing of pregnancy, possibility of oocyte or embryo cryopreservation, and prenatal genetic testing. Those without functional ovaries can achieve pregnancy via oocyte or embryo donation.[12] HRT is required to increase the uterus size and improve its blood flow. HRT should be given for 1 to 2 years before oocyte or embryo transfer.[12] In 1984, the first pregnancy from donated oocytes in a woman with premature ovarian failure was described.[53,54] Although considerable success rates for achieving pregnancies via oocyte donation in women with TS have been reported,[55–57] physicians should not forget the increased risk of hypertensive disorders during pregnancy and preterm deliveries of these individuals.[58,59] It was suggested that the physiologic changes of pregnancy may increase the risk of aortic rupture in the future, after delivery, in patients with TS who made it safely through pregnancy.[60] Pregnant women with TS have a higher risk for fatal aortic dissection or rupture.[12,61] Pregnancy presents a twofold to fivefold increased risk of aortic dissection in patients with TS.[61] The exclusion criteria for pregnancy (spontaneous, assisted, or by oocyte donation) in women with TS are still not well defined, but once pregnancy is achieved it requires strict monitoring and follow-up by a specialized multidisciplinary team.[62] Because of the potential effects of preeclampsia, aortic dissection, and other complications that are increased in TS, patient education and cardiovascular evaluation before pregnancy is warranted in all patients, particularly in those with spontaneous puberty and eventual spontaneous pregnancy.[63] In-depth counseling and strict up-to-date guidelines are essential for appropriate care of individuals with TS who desire pregnancy.

Estrogen Therapy in TS

Estrogen deficiency in girls with TS is already evident in infancy. The optimal age to initiate estrogen replacement therapy is still to be determined. Years ago, before the availability of hGH for treatment of short stature, the recommendation was to delay estrogen replacement therapy until 15 years of age to prevent early epiphyseal fusion and increasing adult height. Because of the theoretical deleterious effects of delaying sexual development, several studies evaluated whether earlier initiation of very small dose of estrogen may improve height velocity without advancing skeletal maturation. Results from a multicenter study conducted in the United States, concluded that the administration of estrogen as early as 8 years of age at variable doses (as low as 25 ng/kg/d) provided no added benefit in adult height gain in patients with TS.[34]

Recent publications suggest that the previously used practice of delaying estrogen therapy should be reconsidered. A double-blind, placebo-controlled trial recently published reported that the combination of low-dose estrogen and hGH improved growth and provided other potential benefits of estrogen replacement.[3] The study included 149 girls who were randomly assigned into different treatment groups: placebo, hGH alone (0.1 mg/kg 3 times a week), estrogen alone, or hGH and estrogen. The doses of oral ethinyl estradiol (or placebo) were adjusted for chronologic age and pubertal status. Oral ethinyl estradiol (25 ng/kg/d) was given to girls 5 to 8 years of age and 50 ng/kg/d for those older than 8 years of age. Patients in all treatment groups who were 12 years or older received escalating doses (100 ng/kg/d–800 ng/kg/d) of ethinyl estradiol based on age. The study concluded that the effect on adult height was greater in the hGH plus ethinyl estradiol group by 2.1 cm (0.32 ± 0.17 standard deviation scores [SDS]) when compared with the hGH alone or placebo group. The investigators suggested that the ultralow dose of ethinyl estradiol may have mediated a local increase in responsiveness to IGF-1 and/or a direct effect of hGH (at the skeletal plate). Because it seemed that the ultralow-dose estrogen did not interfere with GH effects, it was suggested that this combination has potential to optimize adult height and also provide improvements in neurocognitive function, behavior, and self-concept.[3] **Table 2** summarizes selected published studies on combined estrogen and hGH therapy and adult height gains in children with TS.[3,28,34,64]

If no spontaneous breast development has occurred by a certain age (possibly by 10–12 yrs) and serum FSH is elevated, estrogen replacement therapy is recommended.[15] The doses of estrogen should be titrated and guided by breast development, LH, FSH, and bone maturation.[65] The preferred preparation is transdermal estradiol (TDE) as a patch or gel, which provides the most physiologic replacement because it avoids first-pass effects on the liver. If TDE cannot be used, oral estradiol or ethinyl estradiol should be considered.[9] TDE patches can be adjusted to administer very low doses to induce and advance puberty.[12,15]

Anabolic Steroids in TS

Anabolic steroids have been used to optimize height in girls with TS. Several trials in the past 2 decades have recommended the addition of a nonaromatizable, weak anabolic steroid such as oxandrolone (Ox) to hGH. Although there is a general consensus that anabolic steroids accelerate growth velocity, its use has been controversial. In the past, studies have suggested that the combination of hGH and Ox improved height.[66–68] In 2010, a Dutch publication concluded that, compared with hGH plus placebo, the combination of hGH plus Ox at the lower dose of Ox of 0.03 mg/kg/d, resulted in an increase in adult height of 9.5 ± 4.7 cm (SD) compared with 7.2 ± 4.0 (SD) cm observed in the hGH plus placebo group.[69] The lower dose of Ox, although relatively safe, resulted in slight delay of breast development. In contrast, the use of hGH plus the conventional higher dose of Ox (0.06 mg/kg/d), did not significantly improve adult height gain (8.3 ± 4.7 cm) compared with hGH plus placebo (7.2 ± 4.0 cm), but did cause virilization in a larger proportion of patients.[69] Another report indicated that the use of Ox (0.06 mg/kg/d) at mean age of 12 ± 1.7 years in hGH-treated girls with TS, increased growth velocity and adult height after 4 years of treatment; the difference in height and height SDS from baseline was greater in the hGH plus Ox versus the hGH plus placebo groups (26.2 ± 6.7 vs 22.2 ± 5.1 cm).[70] A study conducted in the UK (n = 82) used doses of Ox of 0.05 mg/kg/d (maximum of 2.5 mg) and demonstrated that Ox did increase adult height by 4.6 cm compared with the placebo group.[71] The use of Ox at different dose regimens in conjunction with hGH

Table 2
Studies on combined estrogen and GH therapy and adult height gain in TS

Study	Oral Estrogen Treatment	Cohort	N	Chronologic Age (Baseline) (Y) (Mean ± SD)	Adult Height Attained in SD (Average Gain Over Projected Height, cm)
Ross et al,[3] 2011	Ultralow dose E: Age 5–8 y: 25 ng/kg/d Age 8 y: 50 ng/kg/d Age ≥12 y: escalating doses of 100 ng/kg/d–800 ng/kg/d	A: Double placebo[a] B: E + PL C: hGH (0.1 mg/kg × 3/wk) + PL D: E + hGH	A: 33 B: 37 C: 34 D: 33	A: 7.5 ± 2.3 B: 8.5 ± 2.7 C: 8.2 ± 2.6 D: 9.3 ± 2.5	A: −2.81 ± 0.85 B: −3.39 ± 0.74 C: −2.29 ± 1.10 D: −2.10 ± 1.02
Van Pareren et al,[28] 2003	Childhood low dose E: 5 µg of 17β-estradiol (~0.05 µg/kg/d) in 1st 2 y; 7.5 µg/kg/d in 3rd y 10 µg/kg/d thereafter	A: hGH (4 IU/m²/d) B: hGH (1st y 4 IU/m²/d; thereafter 6 IU/m²/d) C: hGH (1st y 4 IU/m²/d, 2nd y 6 IU/m²/d, thereafter 6 IU/m²/d) (E treatment in each group (A–B) was started after subject reached age 12 y)	A: 19 B: 20 C: 21	A: 6.5 ± 1.9 B: 6.9 ± 2.3 C: 6.5 ± 2.4	A: −1.6 ± 1.0 B: −0.7 ± 1.0 C: −0.6 ± 1.0
Quigley et al,[34] 2002	Childhood low dose E: Age 8 – ≤10 y: 25–50 ng/kg/d Age 10 – ≤12 y: 67–100 ng/kg/d Age ≥12 y: 160–200 ng/kg/d	A: hGH (0.27 mg/kg/wk) + PL B: hGH (0.27 mg/kg/wk) + E C: hGH (0.36 mg/kg/wk) + PL D: hGH (0.36 mg/kg/wk) + E E: Double placebo[a]	A: 15 B: 24 C: 38 D: 22	A: 9.7 ± 2.7 B: 9.6 ± 2.7 C: 9.8 ± 2.9 D: 9.9 ± 2.9	A: −2.2 ± 1.0[b] B: −2.7 ± 1.0[a] C: −1.9 ± 1.0[a] D: −2.2 ± 1.0[a]
Chernausek et al,[64] 2000	Conjugated E: 0.3 mg/d × 6 mo, the increased to 0.625 mg/d	hGH (0.375 mg/kg/wk) A: E start at 15 y B: E start at 12 y	A: 26 B: 29	A: 9.4 ± 0.9 B: 9.6 ± 1.0	A: (8.4 ± 4.3 cm) B: (5.1 ± 3.6 cm)

Abbreviatons: E, estradiol; N, number of patients with Turner syndrome; PL, placebo.
[a] Placebo injection plus childhood oral placebo.
[b] Adult height in (n = 99) subjects whose bone age was at least ≥14 y at the last observation.

in TS has produced variable gains in adult height. It is important to consider the benefit-to-risk ratio before adding Ox to hGH treatment of growth in girls with TS.

Gastrointestinal and Hepatic Disease in TS

There is an increased risk of celiac disease in women with TS.[12,19] The recommendation is to measure tissue transglutaminase IgA antibodies beginning at 4 years of age and subsequently repeat every 2 to 5 years.[12] Individuals with TS also have an increased risk of developing ulcerative colitis.[15] The cause is unclear, but X-chromosome abnormalities seem to play a role in the pathogenesis of inflammatory bowel disease.[19] An increased susceptibility was reported in women with the isochromosome Xq karyotype.[19] Several reports have documented an increased risk for bleeding from intestinal telangiectasia in women with TS.[19,72,73] Although abnormal liver function tests with elevated levels of γ- glutamyl transferase, alanine amino transferase, aspartate amino transferase, and alkaline phosphates have been reported, there was no progression to overt hepatic disease.[5,74] Abnormalities reported include regenerative nodular hyperplasia, hepatic steatosis, billiary lesions, and portal hypertension.[12]

Renal Disorders in TS

Congenital anomalies of the kidney are documented in approximately 30% of patients with TS.[12] Although, renal function is normal, urinary tract infection related to obstruction occur frequently.[12] Because of the risk of hypertension from renovascular abnormalities, it is recommended that all patients with TS have a renal ultrasound at diagnosis and continued monitoring for possible progressive renal impairment and hypertension.[19]

Thyroid Disorders in TS

The most common manifestation of autoimmunity in TS is Hashimoto thyroiditis.[12] The incidence of autoimmune thyroid disease increases with age reaching a peak around 15 years.[19,75] Approximately 83% of TS females with karyotype 46, Xi (Xq), with or without mosaicism, have positive thyroid autoantibodies compared with 41% of 45, X females and 14% of females with other karyotypes.[19,76] It is unclear why individuals with TS are predisposed to autoimmunity. It has been reported that ovarian insufficiency and lack of a second normal X chromosome are associated with an increased development of Hashimoto thyroiditis and other autoimmune disorders.[77] Annual evaluation of thyrotropin and thyroid auto antibodies beginning at age10 years was recommended.[19]

Psychological and Educational Issues in TS

Most individuals with TS are of normal intelligence, although patients with a small ring X-chromosome have increased risk of mental retardation.[12,78] Individuals with TS often experience cognitive impairments in areas of mathematics, visual-spatial function, executive function and specific aspects of language (eg, verbal fluency, complex syntactic knowledge, articulation).[79,80] The cognitive impairments are reported to reflect changes in areas of the brain including the parietal lobe, prefrontal cortex, and the aymgdala.[81–83] Memory, processing speed, and motor skills are influenced by estrogen deficiency and has improved on replacement therapy.[84] Genetic studies have mapped the visuospatial deficits to the PAR 1 of Xp22.3.85.[84,85]

More recent investigations have looked at behavior interventions to help improve performance in individuals with TS.[86] To investigate training effects on performance as well as brain function in a group of children with TS at risk for math difficulties and altered development of math-related brain networks, a study using an adaptive, computerized program that focused on general problem-solving skills was designed.[86] The results indicated significantly increased basic math skills (eg, calculation, processing speed, cognitive flexibility, and visual-spatial processing skills).

In individuals with complete X-monosomy, there is exclusive expression of gene products from a single X-chromosome in each active cell that is either paternally or maternally inherited.[87] This particular pattern of expression allows for studying the effects of genomic imprinting on cognition. Genomic imprinting is a process by which genes are preferentially activated depending on their paternal origin. A prospective study on the impact of genomic imprinting on neurocognitive abilities and social functioning in young girls with TS found no effects of genomic imprinting on standardized measures of cognition.[87] Overall, the data suggested that, although some aspects of the neuropsychological profile of TS could be influenced by epigenetic factors, the sociocognitive phenotype associated with TS was not modulated by genomic imprinting.[87] It did, however, imply that there were genomic imprinting effects on the X-chromosome that affected visual-perceptual reasoning in individuals with TS. Further studies are needed to confirm these findings because previous studies reported conflicting results regarding imprinting effects on some physical and cognitive characteristics of TS.[88,89]

Screening for Associated Comorbidities in TS

Because there is a high rate of related morbidities in individuals with TS, the recommendation is for routine screening for cardiac and celiac diseases, liver dysfunction, dyslipidemia, hearing, and psychological and educational issues.[20] Patient education and early screening during childhood can help improve overall adherence to recommended care. A joint effort between primary and subspecialty care physicians could improve the screening and follow-up in individuals with TS.

NS

NS is a common autosomal dominant disorder with an estimated incidence of 1 per 1000 to 2500 live births, with no gender predominance.[90] NS is characterized by postnatal short stature, congenital heart disease, early feeding difficulties, mild learning disabilities, characteristic facial dysmorphisms, low posterior hairline, webbed neck, and chest deformities. Distinctive facial features include down- slanting palpebral fissures, ptosis, hypertelorism, and low-set posteriorly rotated ears. Additional features include cryptorchidism, lymphatic vessel abnormalities, and hematological abnormalities.[91,92]

The most common congenital heart defect is pulmonary valve stenosis (50%–62%).[93] Hypertrophic cardiomyopathy found in 20% to 30% of individuals can be congenital or may develop in childhood.[93] Diagnosis of NS is mainly based on clinical findings; however, more recently, various genetic mutations have been identified in approximately 61% of the patients.[94]

Autoimmunity in NS

Thyroid antibodies are commonly found in NS, but the development of hypothyroidism is not greater than in the general population.[94,95] Other reported autoimmune conditions in individuals with NS include systemic lupus erythematosus and celiac disease; however, their frequency is unknown.[96–99]

Renal and Genitourinary Anomalies in NS

Renal anomalies are reported to occur in 10% to 11% of individuals with NS and include solitary kidney, renal pelvis dilation, and duplicated collecting system.[94,98]

All individuals should have renal ultrasound at diagnosis and repeat tests depending on the initial findings. If there is a structural abnormality, individuals with NS are at increased risk for urinary tract infections. Antibiotic prophylaxis may raise concern for hydronephrosis and/or recurrent urinary tract infections.[94] Cryptorchidism occurs in 80% of boys and surgical orchiopexy is recommended by 1 year of age if testicles remain undescended at that time. Fertility does not seem to be affected in females.[94] Recent studies suggest that cryptorchidism may not be the main contributing factor; instead Sertoli and Leydig cell dysfunction may play a role in the impairment of testicular function in males with NS. This impairment contributed to the delayed puberty, undescended testes, or infertility described in males with NS.[100]

Bleeding Disorders in NS

There is a variety of hematological abnormalities seen in NS. The hematologic abnormalities found in individuals with NS include thrombocytopenia, platelet dysfunction, von Willebrand disease, and coagulation factor deficiencies.[92] The recommendations include obtaining screening complete blood cell count with differential and prothrombin time and/or activated partial thromboplastin time at diagnosis and, if the initial screen was performed in infancy, after 6 to 12 months of age.[94] The cause of thrombocytopenia is reported to be secondary to decreased megakaryocytes. Clotting factor deficiencies are a common problem in NS. Factor XI deficiency is the most common deficiency seen in NS.[92,101] Reports indicate that there may be an interaction with the gene that causes NS and the regulation of other genes involved in the coagulation pathway.[101] Individuals can have symptoms that are often mild and include bruising, epistaxis, and menorrhagia. However, bleeding with surgical procedures can be significant. It is important for physicians to be aware of the hematological abnormalities seen in NS that, if present, should prompt a more extensive work up. Also, prior knowledge of a homeostatic abnormality in patients with NS can be helpful with patients who undergo invasive procedures that could be improved with better management if bleeding occurs.

Short Stature in NS

About 50% to 70% of individuals with NS have short stature.[94] In contrast to patients with TS, intrauterine growth is normal in NS. In childhood, mean height usually tacks along the third percentile, after which it usually declines progressively when delayed puberty and attenuated pubertal growth spurt occur.[102] There have been conflicting reports on GH secretory dynamics in NS ranging from normal to subnormal spontaneous GH secretion.[103,104] This inconsistency seems to reflect the heterogeneity of this condition. Although the cause of short stature in children with NS is unclear, hGH therapy has been shown to improve growth rates.[5,105–107]

The genetics of NS was poorly understood until recently. The genes causing NS encode members of the RAS-MAPK signal transduction pathway. Missense mutations in the protein tyrosine phosphatase nonreceptor type 11 gene (PTPN11) have been identified.[90] PTPN11 was reported to be the first molecular cause of NS, accounting for approximately 30% to 60% of cases.[90,107] Several other genes were identified, including Kirsten retrovirus-associated DNA Sequences (KRAS), v-raf-1 murine leukemia viral oncogene homolog 1 (RAF1), and Son of Sevenless, homolog 1 (SOS1).[107–110] Rare cases of NS or NS-like disorders have mutations in genes that include NRAS, SHOC2, and CBL.[111] Although genetic testing is available to aid in the diagnosis of NS, because all patients with NS have an identifiable mutation, clinical diagnosis remains essential.

PTPN11 mutation-positive patients have a higher prevalence of short stature than PTPN11-negative patients. NS individuals can carry a heterozygous mutation of the nonreceptor-type protein tyrosine phosphatase, Src homology region 2-domain phosphatase-2 (SHP2), encoded by PTPN11, which plays a role in GH receptor signaling. Mild GH-resistance owing to a postreceptor signaling defect was suggested to be a contributing factor in the growth failure of patients with PTPN11 mutation.[112–114]

Studies on adult height in patients with NS not treated with GH have reported that mean adult height ranged from 161 cm in males (n = 9) and 150.5 cm in females (n = 19)[115] to 162.5 cm in males (n = 20) and 152.7 cm in females (n = 13).[116] A later NS study from the United Kingdom, reported a mean adult height of 169.8 cm in males (n = 18) and 153.3 cm in females (n = 25).[117] Using the Center of Disease Control and Prevention (CDC) standards, it was reported that adult heights in NS (n = 73) were below the third percentile in 38% of males (CDC standards <163.2 cm) and 54.5% of females (CDC standards <151 cm).[118]

GH Treatment in NS

In 2007, the FDA approved GH for treatment of short stature in children with NS. Although trials with hGH therapy have indicated improvement in their growth velocity, the effect was of short duration (**Table 3**).[4–7,119] A long-term study in patients with NS reported that treatment with hGH for up to 6 years of age resulted in an increase in height velocity and height SDS (mean increment in adult height was 3.1 cm).[4] However, a waning effect was noted after 3 years of hGH treatment and only a few patients improved their height prediction by greater than 5 cm. In contrast, a more recent registry-based study (American Norditropin Studies: Web-enabled Research [ANSWER] program) assessing the short-term and long-term effects of hGH therapy in 120 patients with NS treated for up to 4 years, reported an improvement in their height SDS from −2.6 at start of treatment (n = 120) to −1.66 by the end of 3 years of hGH therapy (n = 31) and to 1.32 at the end of 4 years (n = 17).[120] A gain in adult height of 0.6 to 2.0 SDS (4–13 cm) was reported in a small study.[121] An increase of +1.3 (−0.2 to +2.7, SDS) in 29 children with NS with and without the PTPN11 mutation was reported by other investigators.[6] A prospective, uncontrolled, observational study in 18 children with NS evaluating the influence of genotype on the efficacy of hGH therapy reported an increase in height SDS from −2.8 ± 0.9 before start of hGH therapy to −2.0 ± 0.9 12 months later (P<.001).[119] No significant changes in height SDS, height velocity, and serum IGF-1 level were noted between children with and those without PTPN11 mutations. Prospective longer duration studies are required to determine the long-term effects of hGH on height of individuals with NS and elucidate whether a connection exists between the response to hGH therapy and genotype.

GH and Cardiac Function in NS

Because cardiac defects are prevalent in NS, there have been concerns regarding hGH therapy and possible alteration of cardiac function, specifically the development or worsening of left ventricular hypertrophic cardiomyopathy. Earlier reports have shown no changes in cardiac status in individuals with NS treated with hGH.[122–124] A review of the prevalence of cardiac defects and the effects of hGH on the heart of individuals with NS reported no negative effects of hGH therapy, especially on ventricular wall thickness.[125] Because of the limited data available and the high prevalence of cardiac defects in NS, cardiac function should be monitored regularly by clinical examination and ECHO during hGH therapy.[123,125]

Table 3
Studies on GH therapy and adult height gain in children with NS

Study	hGH-Treated Patients (n)	Mean Age of Start (y)	Height SDS[a] At Baseline (Mean)	Initial hGH Dose (mg/kg/wk)	Mean Treatment Duration (y)	Height SDS Gain[b] (From Baseline to Adult Height)
Kirk et al,[4] 2001	66	12.1 (8–15)	−3.1 (−4 to −2)	0.245	5.3 (2–8)	0.6 (0.8)[a]
Osio et al,[5] 2005	18	8.2 (3–14)	−2.9 (−4 to −2)	0.231/0.042	7.5 (4–12)	1.7 (0.4–0.3) 1.7 (0.5–3.1)[a]
Noordam et al,[6] 2008	29	11.0 (6–18)	−2.8 (−4.1 to −1.8)	0.35	6.4 (3–10.3)	1.3 (−0.6–2.4) 1.3 (−0.2 to 2.7)[a]
Raaijmakers et al,[7] 2008	24	10.2	−3.3	0.245	7.6 (4–12)	0.97 (0.6)[a]
Choi et al,[119] 2012	18	8.3 (4.4–13.2)	−2.8 (−5.0 to 1.8)	0.42	1.0	0.8

[a] According to national standards.
[b] According to Noonan standards.

Cancer Risk in NS

The RAS-MAPK pathway is well known for its role in oncogenesis.[126,127]

Patients with NS have a predisposition for leukemia and certain solid tumors.[128] Somatic missense mutations in PTPN11 have been found in approximately one-third of isolated juvenile myelomonocytic leukemia and other myeloproliferative disorders.[127,129] In patients with NS, several case reports have suggested a possible increased incidence of solid tumors, specifically neuroblastoma and embryonal rhabdomyosarcoma.[130–135] The increased risk of cancer in individuals with NS who are PTPN11 mutation-positive requires close monitoring to determine whether hGH therapy may further increase their risk for neoplasia.[111,128,136,137]

Psychological and Educational Issues in NS

There are limited data on the psychological and psychiatric characteristics in individuals with NS. In most individuals with NS, intelligence level is within normal range.[91,138] About one-third of the patients with NS have mild mental retardation. Social and communication problems are reported to be impaired in some individuals with NS.[139] Psychiatric disorders are rarely found and have been reported in patients with NS with lower intelligence. Some reported psychiatric syndromes reported in patients with NS include bipolar affective disorder, schizophrenia, autistic disorder, panic disorder, and alexithymia.[91,140]

SUMMARY

TS and NS are systemic diseases requiring a multisystem management approach. Both conditions are associated with an array of genetic, developmental, cardiovascular, and psychosocial issues. Multidisciplinary interventions specifically geared to different chronologic and developmental stages are essential in TS and NS. Guidelines have been established to help in the care and management of TS. A key feature of both conditions is short stature. Based on over 20 years of data from clinical trials[34,36,68,141] the effects of hGH therapy for short stature associated with TS have been well established. Significant height gains over predicted adult height in individuals with TS following hGH therapy and sex steroid replacement have been reported.[28,32,34] In individuals with NS, most of the evidence for the effects of hGH therapy on growth has come from observational studies in small numbers of subjects and without randomization or control groups. Continued clinical trials of the efficacy of various treatments on height changes in patients with TS or NS are essential for informed clinical decisions and appropriate management.

Efforts to provide optimal, personalized health care to individuals with TS or NS are in progress. These include earlier therapy with hGH and introduction of low-dose estrogen in TS. In individuals with NS, prospective and longer duration studies are still required to determine the long-term effects of hGH on adult height. Research on the effects of hGH therapy on body composition, body mass index, and glucose tolerance require further investigation. The diagnosis and treatment of the various problems that may arise in individuals with TS and NS require a coordinated, expert multidisciplinary team for optimal care.

REFERENCES

1. Davenport ML, Crowe BJ, Travers SH, et al. Growth hormone treatment of early growth failure in toddlers with Turner syndrome: a randomized, controlled, multicenter trial. J Clin Endocrinol Metab 2007;92(9):3406–16.

2. Linglart A, Cabrol S, Berlier P, et al. Growth hormone treatment before the age of 4 years prevents short stature in young girls with Turner syndrome. Eur J Endocrinol 2011;164:891–7.

3. Ross JL, Quigley CA, Cao D, et al. Growth hormone plus childhood low-dose estrogen in Turner's syndrome. N Engl J Med 2011;364(13):1230–42.

4. Kirk JM, Betts PR, Butler GE, et al. Short stature in Noonan Syndrome: response to growth hormone therapy. Arch Dis Child 2001;84:440–3.

5. Osio D, Dahlgren J, Wikland KA, et al. Improved final height with long-term growth hormone treatment in Noonan syndrome. Acta Paediatr 2005;94: 1232–7.

6. Noordam C, Peer PG, Francois I, et al. Long-term GH treatment improves adult height in children with Noonan Syndrome with and without mutations in protein tyrosine phosphatase, nonreceptor-type 11. Eur J Endocrinol 2008;159:203–8.

7. Raaijmakers R, Noordam C, Karagiannis G, et al. Response to growth hormone treatment and final height in Noonan syndrome in a large cohort of patients in the KIGS database. J Pediatr Endocrinol Metab 2008;21:267–73.

8. Rapaport R. Disorders of the Gonads. In: Kliegman RM, Behrman RE, Jenson HB, et al, editors. Nelson text book of pediatrics. 18th edition. Philadelphia: Saunders Elsevier; 2007. p. 2374–84.

9. Davenport ML. Approach to the patient with Turner syndrome. J Clin Endocrinol Metab 2010;95(4):1487–95.

10. Chacko EM, Rapaport R. Short stature and its treatment in Turner and Noonan Syndromes. Curr Opin Endocrinol Diabetes Obes 2012;19(1):40–6.

11. Papp C, Beke A, Mezei G, et al. Prenatal diagnosis of Turner syndrome. J Ultrasound Med 2006;25:711–7.

12. Bondy CA. Care of girls and women with Turner syndrome: a guideline of the Turner syndrome study group. J Clin Endocrinol Metab 2007;92(1):10–25.

13. Saenger P, Wikland KA, Conway GS, et al. Recommendations for the diagnosis and management of Turner Syndrome. J Clin Endocrinol Metab 2001;86: 3061–9.

14. Hook EB, Warburton D. The distribution of chromosomal genotypes associated with Turner's syndrome: live birth prevalence rates and evidence for diminished fetal mortality and severity in genotypes associated with structural X abnormalities or mosaicism. Hum Genet 1983;84:24–7.

15. Pinsker JE. Turner syndrome: updating the paradigm of clinical care. J Clin Endocrinol Metab 2012;97(6):1–10.

16. Mazzanti L, Cicognani A, Baldazzi L, et al. Gonadoblastoma in Turner syndrome and Y-chromosome-derived material. Am J Med Genet A 2005;135:150–4.

17. Tosson H, Rose SR, Gartner LA. Children with 45, X/46, XY karyotype from birth to adult height. Horm Res Paediatr 2010;74:190–200.

18. Bianco B, Lipay M, Guedes A, et al. SRY gene increases the risk of developing gonadoblastoma and/or nontumoral gonadal lesions in Turner syndrome. Int J Gynecol Pathol 2009;28:197–202.

19. Devernay M, Ecosse E, Coste J, et al. Determinants of medical care for young women with Turner syndrome. J Clin Endocrinol Metab 2009;94:3408–13.

20. Nabhan Z, Eugster E. Medical care of girls with Turner syndrome: where are we lacking? Endocr Pract 2011;17(5):747–52.

21. Bondy CA. Congenital cardiovascular disease in Turner syndrome. Congenit Heart Dis 2008;3:2–15.

22. Elsheikh M, Dunger DB, Conway GS, et al. Turner syndrome in adulthood. Endocr Rev 2002;23:120–40.

23. Elsheikh M, Casadei B, Conway GS, et al. Hypertension is a major risk factor for aortic root dilatation in women with Turner's syndrome. Clin Endocrinol (Oxf) 2001;54:69–73.

24. Nathwani NC, Unwin R, Brook CG, et al. The influence of renal and cardiovascular abnormalities on blood pressure in Turner Syndrome. Clin Endocrinol (Oxf) 2000;52:371–7.

25. Spiliotis BE. Recombinant human growth hormone in treatment of Turner syndrome. Ther Clin Risk Manag 2008;4(6):1177–83.

26. Carel JC, Mathivon L, Gendrel C, et al. Near normalization of final height with adapted doses of growth hormone in Turner's syndrome. J Clin Endocrinol Metab 1998;83:1462–6.

27. Stephure DK, the Canadian Growth Hormone Advisory Committee. Impact of growth hormone supplementation on adult height in Turner syndrome: results of the Canadian randomized controlled trial. J Clin Endocrinol Metab 2005;90:3360–6.

28. Van Pareren YK, de Muinck Keizer-Schrama SM, Stijnen T, et al. Final height in girls with Turner syndrome after long-term growth hormone treatment in three dosages and low dose estrogens. J Clin Endocrinol Metab 2003;88:1119–25.

29. Ranke MB, Partsch CJ, Segni M, et al. Adult height after GH therapy in 188 Ullrich-Turner syndrome patients: results of the German IGLU follow-up study 2001. Eur J Endocrinol 2002;147:625–33.

30. Pasquino AM, Pucarelli I, Segni M, et al. Adult height in sixty girls with Turner Syndrome treated with growth hormone matched with an untreated group. J Endocrinol Invest 2005;28:350–6.

31. Soriano-Guillen L, Coste J, Ecosse E, et al. Adult height and pubertal growth in Turner Syndrome after treatment with recombinant growth hormone. J Clin Endocrinol Metab 2005;90(9):5197–205.

32. Ranke MB, Lindberg A, Chatelain P, et al. Prediction of long-term response to recombinant human growth hormone in Turner syndrome: development and validation of mathematical methods. KIGS International Board. Kabi International Growth Study. J Clin Endocrinol Metab 2000;85:4212–8.

33. Reiter EO, Blethen SL, Baptista J, et al. Early initiation of growth hormone treatment allows age-appropriate estrogen use in Turner's syndrome. J Clin Endocrinol Metab 2001;86:1936–41.

34. Quigley CA, Crowe BJ, Anglin DG, et al, U.S. Turner Syndrome Study Group. Growth hormone and low dose estrogen in Turner syndrome: results of a United States multi-center trial to near-final height. J Clin Endocrinol Metab 2002;87(5): 2033–41.

35. Carel JC, Mathivon L, Gendrel C, et al. Growth hormone therapy for Turner syndrome: evidence for benefit. Horm Res 1997;48:31–4.

36. Sas TC, de Muinck K, Stijen T, et al. Normalization of height in girls with Turner Syndrome after long-term growth hormone treatment; results of a randomized dose-response trial. J Clin Endocrinol Metab 1999;84:4607–12.

37. Hofman P, Cutfield WS, Robinson EM, et al. Factors predictive of response to growth hormone therapy in Turner's syndrome. J Pediatr Endocrinol Metab 1997;10:27–33.

38. Hamelin CE, Anglin G, Quigley CA, et al. Genomic imprinting in Turner syndrome: effects on response to growth hormone and on risk of sensorineural loss. J Clin Endocrinol Metab 2006;91:302–3010.

39. Devernay M, Bolca D, Kerdhjana L, et al. Paternal X-chromosome does not influence growth hormone treatment effects in Turner syndrome. J Clin Endocrinol Metab 2012;97(7):e1241–8.

40. Baxter L, Bryant J, Cave CB, et al. Recombinant growth hormone for children and adolescents with Turner Syndrome. Cochrane Database Syst Rev 2007;(1):CD003887.
41. Quigley CA. Growth hormone treatment of non-growth hormone-deficient growth disorders. Endocrinol Metab Clin North Am 2007;36:131–86.
42. Ross J, Lee PA, Gut R, et al. Impact of age and duration if growth hormone therapy in children with Turner syndrome. Horm Res Paediatr 2011;76:392–9. http://dx.doi.org/10.1159/000333073.
43. Parker KL, Wyatt DT, Blethen SL, et al. Screening girls with Turner syndrome: the national cooperative growth study experience. J Pediatr 2003;143:133–5.
44. Blum WF, Cao D, Hesse V. Height gains in response to growth hormone treatment to final height are similar in patients with SHOX deficiency and Turner syndrome. Horm Res 2009;71:167–72.
45. Bolar K, Hoffman AR, Maneatis T, et al. Long-term safety of recombinant human growth hormone in Turner syndrome. J Clin Endocrinol Metab 2008;93:344–51.
46. Hagen CP, Main KM, Kjaergaar S, et al. FSH, LH, inhibin B and estradiol levels in Turner syndrome depend on age and karyotype: longitudinal study of 70 Turner girls with or without spontaneous puberty. Hum Reprod 2010;25(12):3134–41.
47. Reynaud K, Cortvrindt R, Verlinde F, et al. Number of ovarian follicles in human fetuses with the 45, X karyotype. Fertil Steril 2004;81:1112–9.
48. Modi DN, Sane S, Bhartiya D. Accelerated germ cell apoptosis in sex chromosome aneuploid fetal human gonads. Mol Hum Reprod 2003;9:219–25.
49. Nabhan ZM, Dimeglio LA, Qi R, et al. Conjugated oral versus transdermal estrogen replacement in girls with Turner syndrome: a pilot comparative study. J Clin Endocrinol Metab 2009;94(6):2009–14.
50. Pasquino AM, Passeri F, Pucarelli I, et al. Spontaneous pubertal development in Turner's syndrome. J Clin Endocrinol Metab 1977;82:1810–3.
51. Purushothaman R, Lazareva O, Oktay K, et al. Markers of ovarian reserve in young girls with Turner Syndrome. Fertil Steril 2010;94(4):1557–9.
52. Mortensen KH, Rohde MD, Uldbjerg N, et al. Repeated Spontaneous pregnancies in 45, X Turner syndrome. Obstet Gynecol 2010;115:446–9.
53. Lutjen P, Trounson A, Leeton J, et al. The establishment and maintenance of pregnancy using in vitro fertilization and embryo donation in a patient with primary ovarian failure. Nature 1984;307:174–5.
54. Pados G, Camus M, Van Waesberghe L, et al. Oocyte and embryo donation: evaluation of 412 consecutive trials. Hum Reprod 1992;7(8):1111–7.
55. Salat-Baroux J, Cornet D, Alvarez S, et al. Pregnancies after replacement of frozen-thawed embryos in a donation program. Fertil Steril 1988;49(5):817–21.
56. Khastgir G, Abdalla H, Thomas A, et al. Oocyte donation in Turner Syndrome: an analysis of the factors affecting the outcome. Hum Reprod 1997;12(2):279–85.
57. Foudila T, Soderstrom-Anttila V, Hovatta O. Turner's syndrome and pregnancies after oocyte donation. Hum Reprod 1999;14:532–5.
58. Bodri D, Vernaeve V, Figueras F, et al. Oocyte donation in patients with Turner's syndrome: a successful technique but with an accompanying high risk hypertensive disorders during pregnancy. Hum Reprod 2006;21:829–32.
59. Chevalier N, Letur H, Lelannou D, et al. Materno-fetal cardiovascular complications in Turner Syndrome after oocyte donation: insufficient prepregnancy screening and pregnancy follow-up are associated with poor outcome. J Clin Endocrinol Metab 2011;96:E260–7.
60. Reindollar RH. Turner syndrome: contemporary thoughts and reproductive issues. Semin Reprod Med 2011;29(4):342–52.

61. Karnis M. Catastrophic consequences of assisted reproduction: the case of Turner syndrome. Semin Reprod Med 2012;30:116–22.
62. Mercadal B, Imbert R, Demeestere I, et al. Pregnancy outcome after oocyte donation in patients with Turner's syndrome and partial X monosomy. Hum Reprod 2011;26(8):2061–8.
63. Hadnott TN, Gould HN, Gharib AM, et al. Outcomes of spontaneous and assisted pregnancies in Turner Syndrome: the U.S. National Institutes of Health Experience. Fertil Steril 2011;95(7):2251–6.
64. Chernausek SD, Attie KM, Cara JF, et al. Growth hormone therapy of Turner syndrome: the impact of age of estrogen replacement on final height. Genentech, Inc., Collaborative Study Group. J Clin Endocrinol Metab 2002;85:2439–45.
65. Trolle C, Hjerrild B, Cleeman L, et al. Sex hormone replacement in Turner syndrome. Endocrine 2012;41:200–19.
66. Stahnke N, Keller E, Landy H. Favorable final height outcome in girls with Ullrich-Turner syndrome treated with low-dose growth hormone together with oxandrolone despite starting treatment after 10 years of age. J Pediatr Endocrinol Metab 2002;15:129–38.
67. Rosenfeld RG, Attie KM, Frane J, et al. Growth hormone therapy of Turner's syndrome: beneficial effect on adult height. J Pediatr 1998;132:319–24.
68. Nilsson KO, Albertson-Wikland K, Alm J, et al. Improved final height in girls with Turner's syndrome treated with growth hormone and oxandrolone. J Clin Endocrinol Metab 1996;81:635–40.
69. Menke LA, Sas TC, de Muinck Keizer-Schrama SM, et al. Efficacy and safety of oxandrolone in growth hormone-treated girls with Turner syndrome. J Clin Endocrinol Metab 2010;95(3):1151–60.
70. Zeger MP, Shah K, Kowal K, et al. Prospective study confirms oxandrolone-associated improvement in height in growth hormone-treated adolescent girls with Turner syndrome. Horm Res Paediatr 2011;75:38–46.
71. Gault EJ, Perry RJ, Cole TJ, et al. Effect of oxandrolone and timing of pubertal induction on final height in Turner's syndrome: randomised, double blind, placebo controlled trial. BMJ 2011;342:d1980. http://dx.doi.org/10.1136/bmj.d1980.
72. Rutlin E, Wisloff F, Myren J, et al. Intestinal telangiectasis in Turner's syndrome. Endoscopy 1981;13:86–7.
73. Reinhart WH, Mordasini C, Staubli M, et al. Abnormalities of gut vessels in Turner's syndrome. Postgrad Med J 1983;59:122–4.
74. Roulot D, Degott C, Chazouilleres O, et al. Vascular involvement of the liver in Turner's syndrome. Hepatology 2004;39:239–47.
75. Germain EL, Plotnick LP. Age-related anti-thyroid antibodies and thyroid abnormalities in Turner syndrome. Acta Paediatr Scand 1986;75:750–5.
76. Elsheik M, Wass JA, Conway GS. Autoimmune thyroid disease in women with Turner's syndrome—the association with karyotype. Clin Endocrinol 2001;55:223–6.
77. Bakalov VK, Gutin L, Cheng CM, et al. Autoimmune disease in women with Turner syndrome and women with karyotypically normal primary ovarian insufficiency. J Autoimmun 2012;38:315–21.
78. Van Dyke DL, Wiktor A, Palmer CG, et al. Ullrich-Turner syndrome with a small ring X chromosome and presence of mental retardation. Am J Med Genet 1992;43:996–1005.
79. Murphy MM, Massocco MM, Gerner H, et al. Mathematics learning disability in girls with Turner syndrome or fragile X syndrome. Brain Cogn 2006;61:195–210.
80. Knickmeyer R. Turner syndrome: advances in understanding altered cognition, brain structure and function. Curr Opin Neurol 2012;25(2):144–9.

81. Cutter WJ, Daly EM, Robertson DM, et al. Influence of X chromosome and hormone on human brain development: a magnetic resonance imaging and proton magnetic resonance spectroscopy study of Turner syndrome. Biol Psychiatry 2006;59:273–83.
82. Kesler SR, Garrett A, Bender B, et al. Amygdala and hippocampal volumes in Turner syndrome: a high-resolution MRI study of X-monosomy. Neuropsychologia 2004;42:1971–8.
83. Molko N, Cachia A, Riviere D, et al. Brain anatomy in Turner syndrome: evidence for impaired social and spatial-numerical networks. Cereb Cortex 2004;14:840–50.
84. Gajre MP, Parikh P. Neurocognitive profile of Turner syndrome. Indian Pediatr 2011;48:911.
85. Tartaglia N, Hansen R, Hagerman R. Advances in genetics. In: Odom SL, Horner RH, Snell ME, editors. Handbook of developmental disabilities. New York: Guilford Publications; 2009. p. 98–128.
86. Kesler SR, Sheau K, Koovakkattu D, et al. Changes in fronto-parietal training: preliminary results from a pilot study. Neuropsychol Rehabil 2011;21:433–54.
87. Lepage JF, Hong D, Hallamyer J, et al. Genomic imprinting effects on cognition and social abilities in prepubertal girls with Turner syndrome. J Clin Endocrinol Metab 2012;97(3):E460–4.
88. Bondy CA, Matura LA, Wooten N, et al. The physical phenotype of girls and women with Turner syndrome is not X-imprinted. Hum Genet 2007;121:469–74.
89. Sagi L, Zuckerman-Levin N, Gawlik A, et al. Clinical significance of the parental origin of the X-chromosome in Turner Syndrome. J Clin Endocrinol Metab 2007;92:846–52.
90. Tartaglia M, Mehler EL, Goldberg R, et al. Mutations in PTPN11, encoding the protein tyrosine phosphatase SHP-2, cause Noonan Syndrome. Nat Genet 2001;29:465–8.
91. Verhoeven W, Wingbermuhle E, Egger J, et al. Noonan syndrome: psychological and psychiatric aspects. Am J Med Genet A 2008;146:191–6.
92. Briggs BJ, Dickerman JD. Bleeding disorders in Noonan syndrome. Pediatr Blood Cancer 2012;58:167–72.
93. Martinez-Quintana E, Rodriguez-Gonzalez F, Junquera-Rionda P. Noonan syndrome and different morphologic expressions of hypertrophic cardiomyopathy. Pediatr Cardiol 2012. http://dx.doi.org/10.1007/s00246-012-0422-3.
94. Romano AA, Allanson JE, Dahigren J, et al. Noonan syndrome: clinical features, diagnosis, and management guidelines. Pediatrics 2010;126(4):746–55.
95. Allanson JE. Noonan syndrome. Am J Med Genet C Semin Med Genet 2007;145C(3):274–9.
96. Svensson J, Carlsson A, Ericsson UB. Noonan's syndrome and autoimmune diseases. J Pediatr Endocrinol Metab 2003;16(2):217–8.
97. Alany Y, Balci S, Ozen S. Noonan syndrome and systemic lupus erythematous: presentation in childhood. Clin Dysmorphol 2004;13(3):161–3.
98. Lopez-Rangel E, Malleson PN, Lirenman DS, et al. Systemic Lupus erythematous and other autoimmune disorders in children with Noonan syndrome. Am J Med Genet A 2005;139(3):239–42.
99. Lisbona MP, Moreno M, Orellana C, et al. Noonan syndrome associated with systemic lupus erythematous. Lupus 2009;18:267–9.
100. Ankarberg-Lindgren C, Westphal O, Dahlgren J. Testicular size development and reproductive hormones in boys and adult males with Noonan syndrome: a longitudinal study. Eur J Endocrinol 2011;165:137–44.

101. Bertola D, Carneiro JD, D'Amico EA, et al. Hematological Findings in Noonan Syndrome. Rev Hosp Clin Fac Med Sao Paulo 2003;58(1):5–8.

102. Kirk J. Indications for GH therapy in children. Arch Dis Child 2011. http://dx.doi.org/10.1136/adc.2010.186205.

103. Tanaka K, Sato A, Naito T, et al. Noonan syndrome presenting growth hormone neurosecretory dysfunction. Intern Med 1992;31(7):908–11.

104. Limal JM, Parfait B, Cabrol S, et al. Noonan syndrome: relationships between genotype, growth and growth factors. J Clin Endocrinol Metab 2006;91(1):300–6.

105. Gharib H, Cook DM, Saenger PH, et al. American Association of Clinical Endocrinologists medical guidelines for clinical practice for growth hormone use in adults and children—2003 update. Endocr Pract 2003;9(1):64–76.

106. Romano AA, Dana K, Bakker B, et al. Growth response, near-adult height, and patters of growth and puberty in patients with Noonan syndrome treated with growth hormone. J Clin Endocrinol Metab 2009;94(7):2338–44.

107. Ko JM, Kim JM, Kim GH, et al. PTPN11, SOS1, KRAS, and RAF1 gene analysis, and genotype-phenotype correlation in Korean patients with Noonan syndrome. J Hum Genet 2008;53:999–1006.

108. Roberts AE, Araki T, Swanson KD, et al. Germline gain-of-function mutations in SOS1 cause Noonan syndrome. Nat Genet 2007;39(1):70–4.

109. Razzaque MA, Nishizawa T, Komoike Y, et al. Germline gain-of-function mutations in RAF1 cause Noonan syndrome. Nat Genet 2007;39(8):1013–7.

110. Schubbert S, Zenker M, Rowe SL, et al. Germline KRAS mutations cause Noonan Syndrome. Nat Genet 2006;38(3):331–6.

111. Zenker M. Clinical manifestations of mutations in RAS and related intracellular signal transduction factors. Curr Opin Pediatr 2011;23:443–51.

112. Rohrer T. Noonan syndrome: introduction and basic clinical features. Horm Res 2009;72(Suppl 2):3–7.

113. Binder G, Neuer K, Ranke MB, et al. PTPN11 mutations are associated with mild growth hormone resistance in individuals with Noonan syndrome. J Clin Endocrinol Metab 2005;90(9):5377–81.

114. Turner AM. Noonan syndrome. J Paediatr Child Health 2011. http://dx.doi.org/10.1111/j.1440-1754.2010.01970.x.

115. Witt DR, Keena BA, Hall JG, et al. Growth curves for height in Noonan syndrome. Clin Genet 1986;30:150–3.

116. Ranke MB, Heidemann P, Knupfer C, et al. Noonan syndrome: growth and clinical manifestations in 144 cases. Eur J Pediatr 1988;148:220–7.

117. Shaw AC, Kalidas K, Crosby AH, et al. The natural history of Noonan syndrome: a long-term follow up study. Arch Dis Child 2007;92:128–32.

118. Noonan JA, Raaijmakers R, Hall BD. Adult height in Noonan syndrome. Am J Med Genet 2003;123A:68–71.

119. Choi JH, Lee BH, Jung CW, et al. Response to growth hormone therapy in children with Noonan syndrome: correlation with or without PTPN11 gene mutation. Horm Res Paediatr 2012;77:288–393.

120. Lee PA, Ross J, Germak JA, et al. Effect of 4 years of growth hormone therapy in children with Noonan syndrome in the American Norditropin studies: web-enabled research (ANSWER) program(R) registry. Int J Pediatr Endocrinol 2012;(15). http://dx.doi.org/10.1186/1687-9856-2012-15.

121. Dahlgren J. GH therapy in Noonan syndrome: review of final height data. Horm Res 2009;72(Suppl 2):46–8.

122. Cotterill AM, McKenna WJ, Brady AF, et al. The short-term effects of growth hormone therapy on height velocity and cardiac ventricular wall thickness in children with Noonan's syndrome. J Clin Endocrinol Metab 1996;81(6):2291–7.

123. Noordam C, Draaisma JM, va den Nieuwenhof J, et al. Effects of growth hormone treatment of left ventricular dimension in children with Noonan's syndrome. Horm Res 2001;56:110–3.

124. MacFarlane CE, Brown DC, Johnson LB, et al. Growth hormone therapy and growth in children with Noonan's syndrome: results of 3 years' follow-up. J Clin Endocrinol Metab 2001;86(5):1953–6.

125. Noordam C. Growth hormone and the heart in Noonan syndrome. Horm Res 2009;72(Suppl 2):49–51.

126. Bos JL. Ras oncogene in human cancer: a review. Cancer Res 1989;49:4682–9.

127. Pauli S, Steinmann D, Dittmann K, et al. Occurrence of acute lymphoblastic leukemia and juvenile myelomonocytic leukemia in a patient with Noonan syndrome carrying a germline PTPN11 mutation p.E139D. Am J Med Genet A 2011;158:652–8.

128. Jongmans MC, van der Burgt I, Hoogerbrugge PM, et al. Cancer risk in patients with Noonan Syndrome carrying a PTPN11 mutation. Eur J Hum Genet 2011; 19(8):870–4.

129. Tartaglia M, Niemeyer CM, Fragale A, et al. Somatic mutations in PTPN11 in juvenile myelomonocytic leukemia, myelodysplastic syndromes, and acute myeloid leukemia. Nat Genet 2003;34:148–50.

130. Ljiri R, Tanaka Y, Keisuke K, et al. A case of Noonan's syndrome with possible associated neuroblastoma. Pediatr Radiol 2000;30:432–3.

131. Jung A, Bechthold S, Pfluger T, et al. Orbital rhabdomyosarcoma in Noonan syndrome. J Pediatr Hematol Oncol 2003;25:330–2.

132. Kondoh T, Ishii E, Aoki Y, et al. Noonan syndrome with leukamoid reaction and overproduction of catecholamines: a case report. Eur J Pediatr 2003;162:548–9.

133. Moschovi M, Touliatou V, Papadopoulou A, et al. Rhabdomyosacoma in a patient with Noonan syndrome phenotype and review of the literature. J Pediatr Hematol Oncol 2007;29:341–4.

134. Mutesa L, Pierquin G, Janin N, et al. Germline PTPN11 misssense mutation in a case of Noonan syndrome associated mediastinal and retroperitoneal neuroblastic tumors. Cancer Genet Cytogenet 2008;182:40–2.

135. Bentires-Ali JM, Paez JG, David FS, et al. Activating mutations of the Noonan syndrome-associated SHP2/PTPN11 gene in human solid tumors and adult acute myelogenous leukemia. Cancer Res 2004;64:8816–20.

136. Collett-Solberg PF. Update on growth hormone therapy in children. J Clin Endocrinol Metab 2011;96(3):573–9.

137. Binder G. Response to growth hormone in short children with Noonan syndrome; correlation to genotype. Horm Res 2009;72(Suppl 2):52–6.

138. Allanson JE. Noonan syndrome. In: Cassidy SB, Allanson JE, editors. Management of genetic syndromes. 2nd edition. New York: Wiley-Liss; 2005. p. 385–97.

139. Wood A, Massareno A, Super M, et al. Behavioral aspects and psychiatric findings in Noonan's syndrome. Arch Dis Child 1995;72:153–5.

140. Verhoeven WM, Hendrikx JL, Doorakkers MC, et al. Alexithymia in Noonan syndrome. Genet Couns 2004;15:47–52.

141. van Pareren YK, De Muinck Keizer-Schrama SM, Stijnen T, et al. Effect of discontinuation of long-term growth hormone treatment on carbohydrate metabolism and risk factors for cardiovascular disease in girls with Turner syndrome. J Clin Endocrinol Metab 2002;87:5442–8.

Down Syndrome and Thyroid Function

Evan Graber, DO[a],*, Elizabeth Chacko, MD[a],
Molly O. Regelmann, MD[a], Gertrude Costin, MD[a,b],
Robert Rapaport, MD[a]

KEYWORDS

- Down syndrome • Thyroid function • Euthyroidism • Hypothyroidism

KEY POINTS

- Thyroid dysfunction in children with Down syndrome (DS) can occur as early as birth.
- As children with DS age, their risk for thyroid autoimmunity manifested as autoimmune hypothyroidism or Graves disease increases.
- The optimal timing and method for thyroid screening in children with DS remains controversial. The American Academy of Pediatrics recommends annual screening in this population.
- Consensus is needed to establish working definitions of euthyroidism and mild hypothyroidism in all infants, but especially in those with DS.

Down syndrome (DS), which is the most common chromosomal disorder in liveborn infants, is estimated to occur in approximately 1 in 600 births in the United States.[1] It is most often caused by nondisjunction of chromosomes resulting in trisomy 21. In 4% of patients, DS results from a translocation between material on the long arm of chromosome 21 and material on the long arm of either chromosomes 13, 14, or 15 and in another 1% from a mosaic karyotype in which some cells have 46 chromosomes and others have the trisomy 21 genotype.[2] Children with DS have an increased risk for developmental delay and multiple medical problems, including cardiac, pulmonary, and gastrointestinal anomalies, as well as thyroid abnormalities requiring early and appropriate evaluation and monitoring. Thyroid dysfunction occurs in 4% to 18% of children with DS.[3] This article reviews thyroid abnormalities associated with DS.

CONGENITAL HYPOTHYROIDISM

Congenital hypothyroidism (CH) is one of the most common preventable causes of mental retardation. Its incidence in the general population is estimated to be 1 in

[a] Division of Pediatric Endocrinology and Diabetes, Mount Sinai School of Medicine, 1 Gustave L. Levy Place Box 1616, New York, NY 10029, USA; [b] Keck Medical School, Health Sciences Campus, University of Southern California, 1975 Zonal Avenue, Los Angeles, CA 90089, USA
* Corresponding author.
E-mail address: evan.graber@mountsinai.org

Endocrinol Metab Clin N Am 41 (2012) 735–745
http://dx.doi.org/10.1016/j.ecl.2012.08.008
0889-8529/12/$ – see front matter © 2012 Elsevier Inc. All rights reserved.

2000 to 4000 newborn infants and is believed to be increasing.[4,5] Females are affected twice as often as males.[6,7] Causes of CH include malformation or absence of the thyroid gland, dyshormonogenesis, and maternal iodine deficiency. In patients with DS, the reported incidence of CH is significantly increased, ranging from 28[8] to 35[7] times greater than in the general population ($\sim$1 in 113).

Infants with CH are at increased risk for congenital heart disease, gastrointestinal anomalies, and respiratory distress syndrome when compared with infants without CH.[9] Similarly, infants with DS and CH are at increased risk for other congenital anomalies when compared with infants with DS without CH.[10,11] An increased risk of gastrointestinal anomalies such as duodenal atresia and cardiovascular abnormalities has been reported in children with DS and CH when compared with patients with CH and without DS.[10,11] Likewise, infants with DS diagnosed at birth with gastrointestinal anomalies are 8.6 times more likely to also have CH.[12]

Serum thyroid-stimulating hormone (TSH) values more than 10 mU/L in infants more than 2 weeks of age are considered abnormal, and treatment with thyroid hormone replacement is recommended by the American Academy of Pediatrics (AAP).[6] In infants with DS, determining the need for treatment with thyroid hormone supplementation can be challenging. Although many children with DS have moderately increased serum TSH levels not exceeding 10 mU/L, these values are still significantly greater than in controls.[13] Infants with DS with mildly increased TSH values greater than the upper limit for the laboratory (normal range 0.4–4.0 mIU/L) treated with placebo instead of levothyroxine may have a decrease in TSH over time, but these values continue to remain just more than the upper limits of normal.[14] Results of a study that reported increased TSH levels on filter-paper newborn screening in infants with DS compared with controls (7.0 ± 7.45 mU/L vs 3.9 ± 2.43 mU/L) failed to document an increased risk for developing overt hypothyroidism later in childhood.[15]

Altered thyroxine (T4) concentrations have been reported in infants with DS. When compared with controls, significantly lower T4 concentrations were reported in 1 study.[13] These levels, although at the lower end of the normal range, remained mostly within the normal limits for that laboratory.[13] In the absence of anatomic and biosynthetic defects of the thyroid gland or thyroid autoimmunity, it is unclear whether these altered, but not necessarily abnormal, thyroid function tests have any clinical relevance. It has been suggested that T4 and TSH norms should be adjusted for infants with DS in a fashion similar to the specific growth charts established for these children.[16]

Several mechanisms have been suggested to explain the increased incidence of CH in DS. These mechanisms include an exaggerated response to thyroid-releasing hormone (TRH) stimulation, implying immaturity of the hypothalamic-pituitary axis,[17] inappropriate TSH secretion,[18] TSH insensitivity,[17] and reduced TSH bioactivity, resulting in increased TSH with low-normal T4 levels.[19] None of these mechanisms has been confirmed.[13] Using a radioimmunoassay to analyze cyclic adenosine monophosphate (cAMP) levels, plasma from children with DS and subclinical hypothyroidism was incubated with TSH receptor-transfected cells. No significant difference between the cAMP levels generated by the DS samples and those from euthyroid children without DS was found, suggesting normal TSH bioactivity in children with DS and isolated increased TSH levels.[20]

Because of the variability and usually mild nature of TSH increase and T4 depression in infants with DS, it is often challenging to determine if and when to treat with thyroid hormone supplementation. The concern is that inadequate or late treatment may result in worsening of developmental outcomes in children who are already at risk of being delayed. The argument against treatment is the uncertainty that the minor

TSH and T4 abnormalities have any clinical relevance and thus may not justify lifelong treatment. One randomized, double-blind trial of 196 infants with DS with normal T4-based neonatal thyroid screening (T4 $\geq$0.8 SD for samples tested in 1 day) suggested better developmental outcomes with modest improvements in motor development and growth in those treated with thyroxine for the first 2 years of life compared with their nontreated peers.[21] The implication was that infants with DS and normal thyroid function might benefit from thyroid hormone supplementation. More studies are needed to determine the optimal course of intervention in infants with DS with mildly altered thyroid function[5] and determine whether treatment may be warranted in infants with DS and normal thyroid function.[21]

MILD HYPOTHYROIDISM

Whether children with DS with isolated increases in TSH, but normal thyroid hormone levels, should be diagnosed as having mild hypothyroidism remains unclear (**Tables 1 and 2**). Physicians cannot rely on signs and symptoms suggestive of hypothyroidism such as constipation, dry skin, muscle weakness, fatigue, and weight gain to trigger further investigation, because patients with DS may have these features in the absence of hypothyroidism.[22] The AAP recommended monitoring TSH levels at 6 and 12 months and annually thereafter in children with DS, but the guidelines did not discuss whether or not to treat children with isolated increases of TSH.[3] TRH stimulation testing may be helpful in determining the need for treatment in patients with mildly increased TSH values, but TRH is no longer commercially available in the United States.[4,23] Adherence to monitoring guidelines has been variable throughout the United States and Europe.[1,24,25]

The incidence of mild hypothyroidism in DS ranges between 25% and 32%.[22,26] A study of 320 infants and children with DS reported abnormal thyroid function tests in 90 children (28.1%), of whom 81 (90%) were classified as having compensated hypothyroidism with increased TSH and normal thyroid hormone concentrations. In the compensated hypothyroidism group, TSH levels ranged from 11 to 20 mU/L in 25.3%, whereas the rest had TSH levels between 6 and 10 mU/L. Because of the difficulty in clinically discerning between compensated and decompensated hypothyroidism (those with TSH values more than 20 mU/L) the investigators recommended checking thyroid function every 3 months in patients with compensated hypothyroidism. Treatment was recommended in patients with TSH values between 11 and 20 mU/L.[26] The screening recommendation is in contrast to the currently published AAP guidelines.[3]

Another study of 103 children with DS evaluated their thyroid function first between the ages of 6 and 14 years and again 4 to 6 years later. The results indicated that 5% of children with initially normal thyroid function had on retesting an isolated increase of TSH, whereas 70% of children with an isolated increase in TSH on initial testing had normal thyroid function on retesting. These results suggested that most children with DS and isolated increases in TSH level appeared to have a self-limited course with subsequent normalization. This finding led to question whether the AAP guidelines were too strict and whether the recommendation for annual checking of thyroid function is necessary for many children with DS.[19] Another study of 44 children with DS reported mild increases in TSH levels (6.6–26.8 microunits/mL) in 13 (27%) and spontaneous normalization of TSH in 8 of 10 (80%) of those retested. On follow-up, children with initial increase in TSH values did not differ from those with normal TSH with respect to sex, growth patterns, developmental status, or symptoms of thyroid dysfunction.[11]

Table 1
Comparison of screening recommendations in mild hypothyroidism in children with DS

Authors	n	Definition	% With Mild Hypothyroidism	% Spontaneous Resolution of Mild Hypothyroidism	Screening Recommendations
Bull et al (AAP guideline)[3]	N/A	N/A	N/A	N/A	TSH screen at 6 and 12 mo of age, then annually thereafter
Cutler et al[11]	44	6.6–26.8 microunits/mL	27	80	Routine screening (duration between testing not discussed)
Gibson et al[19]	103	$\geq$6 mU/mL	N/A	70	Thyroid screen every 5 y for patients with initial testing revealing isolated increase of TSH unless symptoms develop
Tuysuz and Beker[26]	320	6–20 mU/L (compensated hypothyroidism)	25	N/A	Thyroid screen annually for patients with normal thyroid functions. Screening every 3 mo for those with compensated hypothyroidism

Table 2
Comparison of findings regarding clinical sequelae of mild hypothyroidism in DS

Authors	n	Definition	Clinical Sequelae of Mild Hypothyroidism
Sharav and Collins[30]	94	TSH >5.7 mU/L	Decreased linear growth, weight gain, and head growth
Selikowitz[31]	101	TSH >3.8 (units not given)	No effect of isolated increases of TSH on growth or intelligence. 40% had spontaneous resolution of increased TSH
Tirosh et al[33]	44	N/A	No improvement in cognitive, social, or physical attributes after 8–14 wk of thyroid hormone replacement for low-borderline thyroid functions

The debate remains regarding the best method for screening children with DS. To avoid the invasive and potentially traumatic nature of venipuncture, it was proposed that capillary TSH, similar to that used in newborn screening programs, be used. Capillary TSH measurements were assessed in 200 children with DS. A TSH level greater than 10 mU/L was considered abnormal. All 15 children with increased TSH values by capillary testing were confirmed by venipuncture and those with markedly raised TSH (36–132 mU/L) were immediately started on treatment with levothyroxine.[27] The investigators concluded that capillary TSH screening was not only feasible but also preferable because it was less invasive. They argued that the decreased sensitivity of capillary screening would result in TSH values less than 10 mU/L being intentionally missed, which would decrease unnecessary referrals of patients with mildly increased TSH (<10 mU/L). These investigators argued that annual screening would be sufficient to diagnose patients with evolving hypothyroidism and that capillary TSH measurements would detect TSH values greater than 10 mU/L.[27] These results and conclusions were confirmed by other studies using capillary TSH screening.[28,29] Although the AAP recommended annual TSH screening in children with DS, it did not specify the method of screening.[3]

It is unclear whether mild hypothyroidism in DS requires treatment. A study of 94 children with DS that monitored the participants' growth along with their thyroid function indicated that linear growth, weight gain, and head growth were all slower in the group of children whose TSH levels were greater than 5.7 mU/L compared with those with TSH values less than 5.7 mU/L (considered the normal cutoff in that study).[30] This finding was in contrast to results from another study, which reported that growth was not affected by isolated increases in TSH and detected no difference in intelligence between the group of children with isolated increase of TSH and those with normal TSH values.[31] Spontaneous resolution of isolated increased TSH levels was documented in 40% of the children studied.[31] Another prospective study performed over 6.8 years reported that 31 of 37 (83.7%) children with DS had intermittent increases of TSH, ranging from 5 to 15 uUI/mL. None of these patients progressed to overt hypothyroidism, suggesting that caution should be used when deciding whether or not to recommend treatment.[32] No significant improvement in cognitive, social, or physical attributes was documented after a short intervention of 8 to 14 weeks of thyroid hormone treatment in a small group of patients with DS and low-borderline thyroid function.[33]

Because zinc is a known cofactor of type II deiodinase, which converts T4 to T3, it has been suggested that zinc deficiency may contribute to mild hypothyroidism in children with DS.[34] A study that measured thyroid function and serum zinc concentrations in 25 children with DS reported lower zinc and higher TSH concentrations when compared with 14 children without DS. Normalization of TSH levels was noted after 4 months of zinc supplementation.[35] In contrast, another study in 16 adolescents with DS failed to detect any improvements in thyroid function with zinc supplementation.[36]

A higher prevalence of thyroid dysfunction was documented in institutionalized adult patients with DS when compared with their noninstitutionalized counterparts, suggesting that perhaps previously undiagnosed thyroid dysfunction might be associated with a greater risk for intellectual impairment.[37] A higher incidence of positive thyroid antibodies and abnormal thyroid function consistent with subclinical hypothyroidism was reported in adults with DS and symptoms of Alzheimer disease compared with unaffected counterparts.[38] These findings reinforce the need for frequent monitoring of thyroid function in individuals with DS to prevent deterioration of cognitive function.

AUTOIMMUNE HYPOTHYROIDISM

Patients with DS are at increased risk of developing autoimmune diseases. Prevalence of celiac disease in this population has been reported to be as high as 5% to 10%,[39] and the risk of type 1 diabetes is 3 times higher than that in the general pediatric population.[40] Likewise, autoimmune hypothyroidism is increased and thyroid antibodies have been reported in 13% to 34% of patients with DS.[41] The characteristics of autoimmune hypothyroidism in children with DS are unique in terms of age of onset and sex distribution. In a study of 85 children with DS, half of those found to have hypothyroidism were diagnosed before age 8 years, but only 1 child had thyroid peroxidase (TPO) antibodies and none had thyroglobulin antibodies.[41] Of those children who were euthyroid before age 8 years, TPO antibodies were present in 2 and thyroglobulin antibodies in 1 other. After age 8 years, 1 or both thyroid antibodies were positive in 11 of 13 hypothyroid children, whereas TPO and thyroglobulin antibodies were increased in 3 and 5 of the euthyroid children, respectively. The investigators concluded that although autoimmune thyroid disease appeared to be uncommon before 8 years of age, it was common in older children and adolescents with DS.[41]

Another study in 38 children with DS reported an 18% incidence of autoimmune thyroiditis before 8 years of age with an equal sex distribution, a finding different from the usual female preponderance seen in the general population. Only 19% of patients with mildly increased TSH levels and increased antibody titers on initial screening had complete normalization of TSH levels and conversion to negative antibody status.[42] An increased prevalence of thyroid autoimmunity in children with DS older than 10 to 12 years was reported compared with younger children with DS.[43,44] Thyroid antibodies have been documented in a few children with DS younger than 1 year (5, 8, and 15 months).[11,45] Evidence suggested that thyroid autoimmunity in children with DS is uncommon in early childhood and becomes more prevalent in older children and adolescents.[11,41–45]

Abnormal immune function has been reported in individuals with DS.[46] Several studies have tried to determine whether autoimmune thyroid disease in DS may be directly related to genetic variations on chromosome 21, which may be tied to immune function. An association between autoimmune hypothyroidism and the DQA1 0301 allele found on chromosome 6 was reported.[47] The DQA1 allele, which codes for major histocompatibility complex antigens expressed on B cells,[48] has been associated with increased risk for celiac disease[48] and autoimmune thyroiditis.[49] Because of the strong association between the DQA1 0301 allele and autoimmune hypothyroidism in patients with DS, it was suggested that other genes might be involved in promoting autoimmune hypothyroidism in this population.[47] It was postulated that immune regulatory genes on chromosome 21 may be involved in upregulating the DQA1 0301 allele activity, leading to increased autoimmunity.[47] However, no HLA genotype has been documented to be related to thyroid dysfunction or presence of thyroid antibodies in DS.[43,50]

The autoimmune regulatory gene (AIRE-1) located on chromosome 21 has been implicated as a potential candidate gene that may contribute to autoimmune thyroid disease in DS. AIRE is a transcription factor that is involved in regulating normal immune function, and mutations in this gene have been connected to polyendocrine syndrome type 1 (APS-1).[51] Although this syndrome is typically characterized by primary hypoparathyroidism, adrenocortical failure, and mucocutaneous candidiasis, 2% to 13% of affected patients have been reported to also have autoimmune thyroid disease.[52] A report of a child with DS and apparent thyroid hormone resistance suggested that an altered or modified AIRE-1 could have been responsible for the thyroid hormone resistance and potentially for thyroid autoimmunity.[53] The possibility that the AIRE gene on chromosome 21 may be involved in increased autoimmunity in DS has also been suggested in another study. The sera from 48 patients with DS were analyzed for several autoantibodies commonly seen in APS-1. Seven of 48 (14%) patients had increased antibody titers. The investigators suggested that overexpression of AIRE caused by a third copy of chromosome 21 may increase autoimmunity in patients with DS.[54] Although many have hypothesized on the possible relationship between AIRE-1 and thyroid autoimmunity in DS this has not yet been substantiated.

GRAVES DISEASE AND HYPERTHYROIDISM

Graves disease occurs in about 1 in 5000 (0.02%) children in the general population and has a female predominance (**Table 3**).[55] The risk of Graves disease in patients with DS is significantly increased, with a prevalence of 6.55 in 1000 (0.66%).[56] It is easily diagnosed by its clinical symptoms, which are similar to those in the general population.[56,57] Graves disease in the setting of DS occurs predominantly between late childhood and early adulthood and does not seem to have an increased risk for females, as usually seen in the general population.[56]

Debate continues on how best to treat children with DS and hyperthyroidism. Simultaneous presence of antibodies consistent with both Graves disease and autoimmune hypothyroidism has been reported.[58] One study reported that children with DS and hyperthyroidism who had only increased thyroid-stimulating immunoglobulin responded well to propylthiouracil (PTU) therapy, with subsequent normalization of

Table 3 Comparison of treatment recommendations for Graves disease in DS				
Authors	n	Initial Treatment	Relapse Rate After Withdrawal of Medical Treatment (%)	Recommended Initial Treatment
Goday-Arno et al[56]	12	Carbimazole	100	I-123 ablation
DeLuca et al[57]	28	Methimazole	7.1	Methimazole
Bhowmick and Grubb[58]	5	PTU	N/A	PTU

Abbreviation: PTU, propylthiouracil.

thyroid function and remission of the antibodies within 4 years. Those patients with anti-bodies consistent with both Graves disease and autoimmune thyroiditis responded to PTU, with normalization of thyroid function and subsequent development of hypothy-roidism, requiring thyroid hormone replacement.[58]

It was suggested that children with DS and hyperthyroidism should always be treated with radioactive I-131 ablation because of frequent failure to go into remission while on carbimazole for up to 2 years and repeated relapses when taken off carbima-zole.[56,59] In contrast, a lower relapse rate of 7.1% in patients with DS compared with 31.2% in controls was reported by others, with persistent remission after being taken off methimazole in 46.4% of children with DS compared with 26% in controls.[57] Because of the variability in therapy outcomes, treatment should be individualized and all available options considered when recommending treatment of hyperthy-roidism in patients with DS. Each treatment modality has its own risks and benefits; medical treatment may be complicated by poor compliance, whereas radioactive iodine may increase the risk of nonthyroidal malignancy.[60] Surgery is invasive, but may be indicated in refractory cases of Graves disease or when radioactive iodine is not indicated or desired by the patient and family.

SUMMARY

Children with DS are at risk for multiple medical problems. Thyroid dysfunction can occur as early as birth. An increased risk of mild hypothyroidism characterized by iso-lated increases in TSH has been reported. Whereas TSH levels may normalize in a certain percentage of these children, in others the levels may remain slightly increased, with T4 levels at the lower end of normal. As children with DS age, their risk for thyroid autoimmunity manifested as autoimmune hypothyroidism or Graves disease increases.

The optimal timing and method for thyroid screening in children with DS remain controversial. The AAP recommends annual screening in this population. Reports from other studies indicate that thyroid dysfunction may wax and wane over time and suggest that there is little risk in checking thyroid function as infrequently as every 5 years. The need or benefit of treatment of mild hypothyroidism in DS is still unclear. It has been suggested that newer, more sensitive metabolic or physiologic testing modalities should be developed to aid in diagnosing permanent hypothyroidism, especially when faced with difficult cases such as mild and transient hypothyroidism, as is often seen in DS.[61]

Consensus is needed to establish working definitions of euthyroidism and mild hypothyroidism in all infants,[61] but especially in those with DS. Prospective, carefully controlled, long-term studies examining growth and cognitive outcomes in children with DS will allow for evidence-based recommendations for their management. Mean-time, it seems reasonable to propose thyroid hormone replacement therapy in those with persistently abnormal thyroid function tests.

REFERENCES

1. Fergeson MA, Mulvihill JJ, Schaefer GB, et al. Low adherence to national guide-lines for thyroid screening in Down syndrome. Genet Med 2009;11(7):548–51.
2. Descartes M, Carroll AJ. Human genetics: cytogenetics. In: Kliegman RM, Behrman RE, Jenson HB, et al, editors. Nelson textbook of pediatrics. 18th edition. Philadelphia: Saunders Elsevier; 2007. p. 507–8.
3. Bull MJ, Committee on Genetics. Health supervision for children with Down syndrome. Pediatrics 2011;128:393–406.

4. Simpser T, Rapaport R. Update on some aspects of neonatal thyroid disease. J Clin Res Pediatr Endocrinol 2010;2(3):95–9.
5. Rapaport R. Congenital hypothyroidism: an evolving common clinical conundrum. J Clin Endocrinol Metab 2010;95(9):4223–5.
6. Brown RS, Foley T, Kaplowitz PB, et al. Update of newborn screening and therapy for congenital hypothyroidism. Pediatrics 2006;117:2290–303.
7. Roberts HE, Moore CA, Fernhoff PM, et al. Population study of congenital hypothyroidism and associated birth defects, Atlanta, 1979-1992. Am J Med Genet 1997;71:29–32.
8. Fort P, Lifshitz F, Bellisario R, et al. Abnormalities of thyroid function in infants with Down syndrome. J Pediatr 1984;104(4):545–9.
9. Fernhoff PM, Brown AL, Elsas LJ. Congenital hypothyroidism: increased risk of neonatal morbidity results in delayed treatment. Lancet 1987;1(8531):490–1.
10. Gu Y, Harada S, Kato T, et al. Increased incidence of extrathyroidal congenital malformations in Japanese patients with congenital hypothyroidism and their relationship with Down syndrome and other factors. Thyroid 2009;19(8): 869–79.
11. Cutler AT, Benezra-Obeiter R, Brink SJ. Thyroid function in young children with Down syndrome. Am J Dis Child 1986;140:479–83.
12. Jaruratanasirikul S, Patarakijvanich N, Patanapisarnsak C. The association of congenital hypothyroidism and congenital gastrointestinal anomalies in Down's syndrome infants. J Pediatr Endocrinol Metab 1998;11:241–6.
13. Van Trotsenburg AS, Vulsma T, Van Santen HM, et al. Lower neonatal screening thyroxine concentrations in Down syndrome newborns. J Clin Endocrinol Metab 2003;88(4):1512–5.
14. Van Trotsenburg AS, Kempers MJ, Endert E, et al. Trisomy 21 causes persistent congenital hypothyroidism presumably of thyroidal origin. Thyroid 2006;16(7): 671–80.
15. Myrelid A, Jonsson B, Guthenberg C, et al. Increased neonatal thyrotropin in Down syndrome. Acta Paediatr 2009;98:1010–3.
16. Prasher V, Haque MS. Misdiagnosis of thyroid disorders in Down syndrome: time to re-examine the myth? Am J Ment Retard 2005;110(1):23–7.
17. Sharav T, Landau H, Zadik Z, et al. Age-related patterns of thyroid-stimulating hormone response to thyrotropin-releasing hormone stimulation in Down syndrome. AJDC 1991;145:172–5.
18. Gruneiro de Papendieck L, Chiesa A, Bastida MG, et al. Thyroid dysfunction and high thyroid stimulating hormone levels in children with Down syndrome. J Pediatr Endocrinol Metab 2002;15:1543–8.
19. Gibson PA, Newton RW, Selby K, et al. Longitudinal study of thyroid function in Down's syndrome in the first two decades. Arch Dis Child 2005;90:574–8.
20. Konings CH, Van Trotsenburg AS, Ris-Stalpers C, et al. Plasma thyrotropin bioactivity in Down's syndrome children with subclinical hypothyroidism. Eur J Endocrinol 2001;144:1–4.
21. Van Trotsenburg AS, Vulsma T, van Rozenburg-Marres SL, et al. The effect of thyroxine treatment started in the neonatal period on development and growth of two-year-old Down syndrome children: a randomized clinical trial. J Clin Endocrinol Metab 2005;90(6):3304–11.
22. O'Grady MJ, Cody D. Subclinical hypothyroidism in childhood. Arch Dis Child 2011;96:280–4.
23. Rapaport R, Akler G, Regelmann M, et al. Time for thyrotropin releasing hormone to return to the United States of America. Thyroid 2010;20(9):947–8.

24. Carroll KN, Arbogast PG, Dudley JA, et al. Increase in incidence of medically treated thyroid disease in children with Down syndrome after rerelease Of American Academy of Pediatrics health supervision guidelines. Pediatrics 2008;122:e493–8.

25. Varadkar S, Bineham G, Lessing D. Thyroid screening in Down syndrome: current patterns in the UK. Arch Dis Child 2003;88(7):647.

26. Tuysuz B, Beker DB. Thyroid dysfunction in children with Down's syndrome. Acta Paediatr 2001;90:1389–93.

27. Noble SE, Leyland K, Findlay CA, et al. School based screening for hypothyroidism in Down's syndrome by dried blood spot TSH measurement. Arch Dis Child 2000;82:27–31.

28. McGowan S, Jones J, Brown A, et al. Capillary TSH screening programme for Down's syndrome in Scotland, 1997-2009. Arch Dis Child 2011;96:1113–7.

29. Murphy J, Philip M, Macken S, et al. Thyroid dysfunction in Down's syndrome and screening for hypothyroidism in children and adolescents using capillary TSH measurement. J Pediatr Endocrinol Metab 2008;21(2):155–63.

30. Sharav T, Collins RM, Baab PJ. Growth studies in infants and children with Down's syndrome and elevated levels of thyrotropin. AJDC 1988;142:1302–6.

31. Selikowitz MA. Five-year longitudinal study of thyroid function in children with Down syndrome. Dev Med Child Neurol 1993;35:396–401.

32. Faria CD, Ribeiro S, Kochi C, et al. TSH neurosecretory dysfunction (TSH-nd) in Down syndrome (DS): low risk of progression to Hashimoto's thyroiditis. Arq Bras Endocrinol Metabol 2011;55(8):628–31.

33. Tirosh E, Taub Y, Scher A, et al. Short-term efficacy of thyroid hormone supplementation for patients with Down syndrome and low-borderline thyroid function. Am J Ment Retard 1989;93(6):652–6.

34. Thiel R, Fowkes SW. Down syndrome and thyroid dysfunction: should nutritional support be the first-line treatment? Med Hypotheses 2007;69:809–15.

35. Licastro F, Mocchegiani E, Zonnotti M, et al. Zinc affects the metabolism of thyroid hormones in children with Down's syndrome: normalization of thyroid stimulating hormone and of reversal triiodothyronine plasmic levels by dietary zinc supplementation. Int J Neurosci 1992;65:259–68.

36. Marreiro D, de Sousa AF, Nogueira N, et al. Effect of zinc supplementation on thyroid hormone metabolism of adolescents with Down syndrome. Biol Trace Elem Res 2009;129:20–7.

37. Rooney S, Walsh E. Prevalence of abnormal thyroid function tests in a Down's syndrome population. Ir J Med Sci 1997;166(2):80–2.

38. Percy ME, Dalton AJ, Markovic VD, et al. Autoimmune thyroiditis associated with mild "subclinical" hypothyroidism in adults with Down syndrome: a comparison of patients with and without manifestations of Alzheimer disease. Am J Med Genet 1990;36:148–54.

39. Cohen WI. Current dilemmas in Down syndrome clinical care: celiac disease, thyroid disorders, and atlanto-axial instability. Am J Med Genet 2006;142C:141–8.

40. Van Goor JC, Massa GG, Hirasing R. Increased incidence and prevalence of diabetes mellitus in Down's syndrome. Arch Dis Child 1997;77:186.

41. Karlsson B, Gustafsson J, Hedov G, et al. Thyroid dysfunction in Down's syndrome: relation to age and thyroid autoimmunity. Arch Dis Child 1998;79:242–5.

42. Popova G, Paterson WF, Brown A, et al. Hashimoto's thyroiditis in Down's syndrome: clinical presentation and evolution. Horm Res 2008;70:278–84.

43. Zori RT, Schatz DA, Ostrer H, et al. Relationship of autoimmunity to thyroid dysfunction in children and adults with Down syndrome. Am J Med Genet Suppl 1990;7:238–41.

44. Ivarsson SA, Ericsson UB, Gustafsson J, et al. The impact of thyroid autoimmunity in children and adolescents with Down syndrome. Acta Paediatr 1997;86:1065–7.
45. Shalitin S, Phillip M. Autoimmune thyroiditis in infants with Down's syndrome. J Pediatr Endocrinol Metab 2002;15:649–52.
46. Levo Y, Green P. Down's syndrome and autoimmunity. Am J Med Sci 1977;273(1): 95–9.
47. Nicholson LB, Wong FS, Ewins DL, et al. Susceptibility to autoimmune thyroiditis in Down's syndrome is associated with the major histocompatibility class II DQA 0301 allele. Clin Endocrinol 1994;41:381–3.
48. Online Mendelian inheritance in man, OMIM®. Johns Hopkins University, Baltimore (MD). MIM Number: 212750: 6/16/11: World Wide Web URL: Available at: http://omim.org/. Accessed July 19, 2012.
49. Zeitlin AA, Heward JM, Newby PR, et al. Analysis of HLA class II genes in Hashimoto's thyroiditis reveals differences compared to Graves' disease. Genes Immun 2008;9:358–63.
50. McLachlan SM. Editorial: the genetic basis of autoimmune thyroid disease: time to focus on chromosomal loci other than the major histocompatibility complex (HLA in Man). J Clin Endocrinol Metab 1993;77(3):605A–605C.
51. Online Mendelian inheritance in man, OMIM. Johns Hopkins University, Baltimore (MD). MIM Number: 240300: 1/27/12: World Wide Web URL: Available at: http://omim.org/. Accessed July 19, 2012.
52. Dittmar M, Kahaly GJ. Immunoregulatory and susceptibility genes in thyroid and polyglandular autoimmunity. Thyroid 2005;15(3):239–50.
53. Fernandez-Garcia JC, Lopez-Medina JA, Berchid-Debdi M, et al. Resistance to thyroid hormone and Down syndrome: coincidental association or genetic linkage? Thyroid 2012;22(9):973–4.
54. Soderburgh A, Gustafsson J, Ekwall O, et al. Autoantibodies linked to autoimmune polyendocrine syndrome type I are prevalent in Down syndrome. Acta Paediatr 2006;95:1657–60.
55. LaFranchi S. The endocrine system: disorders of the thyroid gland. In: Kliegman RM, Behrman RE, Jenson HB, et al, editors. Nelson textbook of pediatrics. 18th edition. Philadelphia: Saunders Elsevier; 2007. p. 2333.
56. Goday-Arno A, Cerda-Esteva M, Flores-Le-Roux JA, et al. Hyperthyroidism in a population with Down syndrome (DS). Clin Endocrinol 2009;71:110–4.
57. De Luca F, Corrias A, Salerno M, et al. Peculiarities of Graves' disease in children and adolescents with Down's syndrome. Eur J Endocrinol 2010;162:591–5.
58. Bhowmick SK, Grubb PH. Management of multiple-antibody-mediated hyperthyroidism in children with Down's syndrome. South Med J 1997;90(3):312–5.
59. Damle N, Das K, Bal C. Graves' disease in a Down's syndrome patient responds well to radioiodine rather then antithyroid drugs. J Pediatr Endocrinol Metab 2011;24(7–8):611.
60. Bhat MH, Saba S, Ahmed I, et al. Graves' disease in a Down's syndrome patient. J Pediatr Endocrinol Metab 2010;23:1181–3.
61. Rapaport R. Congenital hypothyroidism: expanding the spectrum. J Pediatr 2000;136:10–2.

Growth and Growth Hormone Treatment in Children with Chronic Diseases

Alba Morales Pozzo, MD*, Stephen F. Kemp, MD, PhD

KEYWORDS

- Growth hormone • Short stature • Burns • Short bowel syndrome
- Chronic inflammation • Short bowel syndrome • Cystic fibrosis
- Chronic kidney disease

KEY POINTS

- Growth hormone (GH) is a powerful growth-promoting anabolic hormone that may have further use in treating a number of chronic childhood diseases.
- When used to treat cystic fibrosis, GH may offer stimulation of linear growth, as well as better energy balance.
- Height- and nonheight-related benefits of GH therapy in patients suffering from chronic inflammatory conditions like juvenile idiopathic arthritis (JIA) and Crohn disease (CD) have been reported and will need to be further studied.
- GH should not be used in critically ill patients, since it has been associated with increased mortality in this population.
- The chronic use of glucocorticoids induces a catabolic state that may be ameliorated by the concomitant use of GH in some patients.
- Beneficial effects of GH therapy in conditions like thermal trauma, short bowel syndrome and X-linked hypophosphatemic rickets have been reported and deserve further study.

INTRODUCTION

Growth hormone (GH) was first used to treat a patient in 1958.[1] For the next 25 years, it was available only from cadaver sources, which was of concern because of safety considerations and short supply. In 1985, GH produced by recombinant DNA techniques became available, expanding its possible uses. Since that time there have been three indications approved by the US Food and Drug Administration (FDA) for GH deficiency and 9 indications approved for non-GH deficiency (GHD) states. Numerous clinical trials support its use in children with GHD as well as other disorders associated with growth

Arkansas Children's Hospital, University of Arkansas for Medical Sciences, 1 Children's Way, Little Rock, AR 72202-3591, USA
* Corresponding author.
E-mail address: MoralesAlba@uams.edu

Endocrinol Metab Clin N Am 41 (2012) 747–759
http://dx.doi.org/10.1016/j.ecl.2012.07.001
0889-8529/12/$ – see front matter © 2012 Elsevier Inc. All rights reserved.

endo.theclinics.com

failure. Some of these are chronic diseases, such as chronic renal insufficiency (CRI), while others are genetic disorders, such as Turner syndrome (TS) or Prader-Willi syndrome (PWS), and some are disorders for which the cause of short stature is less clear, such as small for gestational age (SGA) and idiopathic short stature (ISS). Recently, clinical trials investigating GH therapy in other chronic childhood diseases have shown promising results. The following sections will summarize the work of these investigators in specific chronic childhood conditions and will touch briefly on the mechanism by which these conditions cause growth abnormalities in the patients (**Fig. 1**).

GH Therapy in Cystic Fibrosis

Cystic fibrosis (CF) is an autosomal recessive disorder caused by mutation of the CF transmembrane regulator protein, which regulates sodium and chloride transport across epithelial membranes. CF is characterized by viscous secretions of exocrine glands, endocrine pancreas insufficiency, and growth failure and malnutrition. More than 25% of children with CF have been reported to be below the 10th percentile in weight, and almost 30% are below the 10th percentile for height.[2] Since the advent of recombinant GH, there has been interest in using GH to treat the growth issues, as well as to help address some of the nutritional problems relating to their increased energy expenditure. Several studies have suggested that GH therapy in CF increases growth velocity as well as weight.[3,4] A recent evaluation of 10 controlled clinical trials[5] and 8 observational studies[5] showed that in the controlled trials, markers of pulmonary function, anthropometrics, and bone mineralization all appeared to be increased compared with controls. With regard to long-term health issues, such as pulmonary exacerbations, hospitalizations, or mortality, the only significant finding was that GH therapy seemed to reduce the rate of hospitalizations. A recent study of 68 subjects with CF (32 were controls, and 36 received GH for 12 months)[6] demonstrated that GH promoted an increase in growth, weight, lean body mass, lung volume, and lung flow. In addition, it had an acceptable safety profile. Therefore, data for treatment of CF appear promising; however, this indication has not been approved by the FDA.

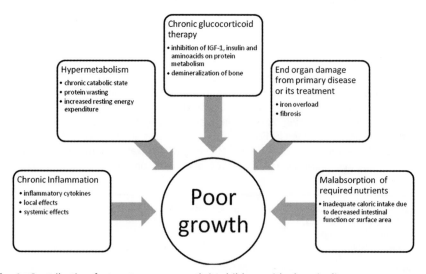

Fig. 1. Contributing factors to poor growth in children with chronic diseases.

GH Therapy in Chronic Inflammation/Chronic Steroid Use

Juvenile idiopathic arthritis

Juvenile idiopathic arthritis (JIA) is also known as juvenile rheumatoid arthritis, Still disease, or juvenile chronic polyarthritis. It is a childhood disease characterized by chronic joint inflammation, pain, and fever, thought to be of autoimmune origin. Systemic disease is the least common form of JIA but results in severe growth impairment, which is worse in patients who require long-term therapy with glucocorticoids. Children with JIA suffer changes in bone development, believed to be caused at least in part by an imbalance of proinflammatory cytokines. Critical cytokines involved in chronic inflammation include: interleukin 1β (IL-1β), tumor necrosis factor α (TNFα), and IL-6.[7] Proinflammatory cytokines are immune-cell derived polypeptides with many target cells and actions; these cytokines bind to specific cell surface receptors, causing effects in gene expression in their target cells. Different cytokines may affect the same transduction pathways in a cell and thus may have cross-over effects among each other. Cytokines may cause localized and systemic effects causing bone abnormalities.

Adult height Standard Deviation Score (SDS) of less than -2 denotes significant short stature and can be found in 11% to 41% of children with JIA, the higher proportion found in patients with the systemic form of the disease.[8,9] Severe general growth retardation has been described in children suffering from systemic JIA, and significant deviation from midparental height seems to be associated with glucocorticoid therapy lasting more than 12 months in these children.[10] Systemic and local effects of the proinflammatory state on the growth hormone–insulinlike growth factor-1 (IGF-1) growth plate axis have been described. Pediatric JIA patients with elevated levels of IL-6 have been found to have reduced circulating levels of IGF-1 and IGF-BP3 with unchanged serum GH levels.[11,12] IL-6 neutralization was found to normalize growth in a murine model of this phenomenon. It is probable that IL-6 reduces IGF-1 en serum by increasing its clearance rate, as IGF-1's half-life is markedly prolonged due to its association in the circulation with IGF-BP3 and amyotrophic lateral sclerosis (ALS).[13] Deleterious local effects of inflammatory cytokines on the growth plate have been previously described, and IL-6 reduces the stimulatory effect of IGF-1 on proteoglycan synthesis in the growth plate.[14] In general, IL-6 affects growth mainly via systemic mechanisms altering GH secretion, and IL-1β and TNF-α are able to directly influence growth plate chondrocyte dynamics as well as linear bone growth.[15]

Between the years of 1979 and 2003, 4 observational drug trials and 1 controlled trial found beneficial effects of GH therapy in children with JIA. GH dosages ranged from 0.1 to 0.46 mg/kg/wk. In the observational studies, significant increases in growth velocity and IGF-1/IGF-BP3 levels were reported in the first year of treatment. The acceleration of linear growth returned to normal within the first year of treatment, and the growth factors elevated levels persisted throughout the time of GH treatment. Results from these therapeutic trials show that GH therapy can decrease the height deficit that occurs during the active phase of JIA, giving rise to a final height that is close to the midparental target height.[16]

Nonheight-related beneficial effects of GH therapy in patients with JIA have been documented. In a recent longitudinal study, muscle and fat cross-sectional areas (CSAs) were measured on a yearly basis until final height in 12 patients with JIA receiving GH therapy. Data were compared with measurements in 13 patients with JIA not receiving GH treatment. Results of this study showed that GH therapy created a normalization and increase of total bone and muscle CSA at final height. Treated patients' fat mass stabilized at the lower limit of normal for healthy children in keeping to the anabolic effect of GH.[17]

Crohn disease

Up to 80% of newly diagnosed children with Crohn disease (CD) have growth failure in their initial presentation.[18] Long-term use of glucocorticoid therapy is often necessary for maintenance of remission in CD, further exacerbating growth delay. Several studies have described multiple benefits of GH therapy in CD. Recently, a randomized controlled trial of GH in 20 pediatric patients with active CD found that the addition of GH to corticosteroid therapy led to an improvement in disease activity, compared with steroid therapy alone. A significant steroid-sparing effect of GH was also noted in this study.[19] Three studies had previously shown benefits of GH therapy in CD.[20–22] Their findings included: an increase in height velocity and bone density in 10 children with CD with an average age of 12.5 years; positive changes in body composition, linear growth, and bone metabolism in corticosteroid-dependent patients with inflammatory bowel disease (in the absence of glucose metabolism deterioration); and amelioration in the clinical severity of the disease in 37 adult patients with CD as measured by a decrease in their CD activity index score after 4 months of GH therapy.

Chronic glucocorticoid use in CD, CFm and JIA—role of GH therapy

Children who suffer from chronic inflammatory diseases like CD and JIA frequently require long-term use of anti-inflammatory agents including glucocorticoids. Chronic use of glucocorticoids produces a chronic catabolic effect on protein metabolism and body composition by inhibiting the stimulatory actions of IGF-1, insulin, and amino acids on protein synthesis.[23] On the other hand, GH is an effective anabolic and growth-promoting agent in vivo and in vitro. As mentioned in the previous section, GH use in children with CD has a beneficial metabolic effect. GH was able to counteract some of the negative metabolic effects caused by long-term GCs use; bone calcium accretion was increased, as was lean body mass with a decrease of adiposity.[21] Protein metabolism, growth, and clinical status were also improved after GH treatment in children suffering from CF requiring chronic glucocorticoid use.[24,25] A 3-year trial of GH therapy in children with JIA and steroid dependency revealed significant improvement in mean height standard deviation score and mean height velocity in treated patients when compared with untreated children.[9] The authors found GH treatment to be well tolerated, with fasting insulin levels significantly increased in GH-treated patients but unchanged fasting glycemia. Chronic use of glucocorticoids can cause a severe catabolic state that may be at least partially ameliorated by concomitant use of GH therapy.

Hypermetabolism/Thermal Injury

Critically ill patients

In the 1990s there was interest in treating catabolic patients with GH. Two large placebo-controlled studies were undertaken in intensive care patients with heart or abdominal surgery, trauma, or acute respiratory failure. Both studies were concluded early when an interim evaluation of the data demonstrated that the mortality rate in both studies was significantly higher in those patients receiving GH (41.9% vs 19.3%).[26,27] It is now the recommendation not to treat critically ill patients with GH, especially patients with an active infection or sepsis.

Burns

GH was used soon after recombinant GH was available to increase donor site healing in patients with severe burns.[28] Lal and colleagues[29] demonstrated that patients receiving large doses of GH (0.2 mg/kg/d) had length of stay decreased by approximately 14 days. Because of concern about increased mortality seen in critically ill adults, they compared mortality rates between these patients and a control group. Mortality rates for those receiving GH were not different from controls. In addition to increasing donor site healing,

GH therapy may alter healing of the injury from the burn. After the acute inflammatory response caused by severe burn trauma, persistent metabolic abnormalities give rise to a catabolic state characterized by protein wasting, increased resting energy expenditure, and protein release from fat and muscle stores that may persist many months after the thermal injury has healed. Such a hypermetabolic state correlates directly with morbidity and mortality. GH is a potent anabolic agent with the potential to counteract the negative metabolic effects of burn trauma, but its use has been associated with increased mortality in critically ill patients in the past. Administration of recombinant human GH (rhGH) has been shown to decrease whole body catabolism,[30] improve muscle protein synthesis,[31,32] improve wound healing[33] and immune function,[34] and promote linear growth.[35] Proven deleterious effects of rhGH therapy in critically ill patients such as increased serum levels of glucose, free fatty acids, and triglycerides could contribute to increased morbidity and mortality in this population.[27] Recently, a prospective randomized control trial of rhGH used in combination with propranolol in severely burned children showed that this combination attenuated hypermetabolism and inflammation without the adverse side effects found with rhGH therapy alone.[36] More recently, a large prospective randomized single-center controlled clinical trial in pediatric patients with massive burns enrolled between 1998 and 2007 demonstrated the following results: rhGH significantly improved growth and lean body mass while attenuating hypermetabolism; GH-treated patients had increased levels of serum GH, IGF-1 and IGF-BP3, and percent body fat content was decreased. Additionally, resting energy expenditure improved with GH treatment, and long-term administration of GH significantly improved scarring at 12 months after the burn.[37] The authors concluded that long-term treatment with GH enhanced recovery of severely burned pediatric patients.

Short Bowel Syndrome

Short Bowel Syndrome (SBS) in children results from inadequate intestinal adaptation to massive resection of intestine, most commonly due to necrotizing enterocolitis, intestinal atresias, and midgut volvulus. Ideally, the remnant intestine shows a critical adaptive response by increasing protein, DNA content, villus height, and crypt depth, in an effort to compensate for lost absorptive and digestive capacities. The degree to which the intestine can adapt to this loss is a critical determinant for subsequent nutrient absorption needed for optimal growth and development in the child. The GH receptor can be found throughout the intestinal layers and its epithelium,[38] which has led investigators to propose GH as a direct stimulant of intestinal growth. Human clinical trials involving GH treatment of adults with SBS have had mixed results in the past. Most studies have demonstrated GH therapy in combination with dietary modification and the addition of glutamine have helped patients gain body weight and mass.[39,40] Some studies in adults and children show GH facilitates weaning off parenteral nutrition.[39,41] Clinical trials of GH therapy in SBS show that patients with 70 to 100 cm of remnant bowel and without an intact colon have the greatest benefit from GH, as this group had the greatest rate of complete discontinuation of parenteral nutrition.[42]

GH Therapy in Hypophosphatemic Rickets

Hypophosphatemic rickets includes hypophosphatemic rickets, autosomal dominant hypophosphatemic rickets, autosomal recessive hypophosphatemic rickets, tumor-induced osteomalacia, and fibrous dysplasia. All of these disorders are characterized by low levels of serum phosphate, which does not allow good function of the mature osteoblasts, leading to poor linear growth. X-linked hypophosphatemic rickets (XLHR) is the most common form of hypophosphatemic rickets. Conventional therapy has included supplementation with oral phosphate and vitamin D. Growth response to conventional therapy is disappointing, in part because oral phosphate is unpalatable, and there is often noncompliance. Since the advent of recombinant GH, there has been interest in investigating whether GH would increase the growth response (and ultimately final height) in patients with this disorder. Such studies have been limited because of the small numbers of subjects studied (due to the rare nature of the disorder). Saggese and colleagues[43,44] studied 12 subjects, of whom 6 received conventional therapy plus GH and 6 received only conventional therapy. They concluded that those receiving GH showed an increase in height Z-score, growth velocity Z-score, and predicted final height, along with increases in serum phosphate, bone markers, bone alkaline phosphatase, parathyroid hormone, 1,25-hydroxy vitamin D, and bone mineral density. Reusz and colleagues[45] similarly treated 6 children with XLHR with GH, and showed an increase in height Z-score and a slight increase in serum phosphate. However, there was no control group. Wilson[46] reviewed 7 clinical trials and concluded that GH appeared to increase growth velocity, although there were no final height data. He did note that GH therapy appeared to be safe. A subsequent study[47] did report final height data in a study of 12 patients with XLHR (6 treated with conventional therapy plus GH, and 6 treated only with conventional therapy). These results showed that GH treatment for as long as 10 years was associated with an increase in height standard deviation score of 1 SD at the time final height was achieved. Another analysis of published data by Huiming[48] found that of the 5 published trials they found, only 1 met their inclusion criteria. This trial included only 5 participants, but it did show an increase in height standard deviation score with GH. However, their conclusion was that there was no conclusive evidence that GH therapy in XLHR increased linear growth or changed mineral metabolism, renal function, bone mineral density, or body proportions. However, GH therapy did appear to be safe. At this point, it seems clear that treatment with GH is safe, but it is not yet possible to say whether GH treatment is truly effective, or if there is a growth response, how large an increase in final height there would be. More investigation with appropriate controls and greater numbers of subjects is necessary before it can be determined that GH is of benefit in this condition.

Beta-Thalassemia Major and GH Therapy

Beta-thalassemia major is a severe congenital hematologic abnormality that requires regular blood transfusion therapy with the goal of keeping the patient's hemoglobin level above 9 mg/dL. Chelation therapy is used to attempt iron overload prevention. Endocrine organs are particularly susceptible to iron overload. Growth axis and pubertal abnormalities are well described consequences of beta-thalassemia and its treatment.[49–55] The pathogenesis of poor growth and delayed puberty is multifactorial (growth hormone deficiency, liver disease, chronic anemia, zinc and folic acid deficiencies, hypogonadism, iron overload), but the pattern of abnormal growth seen in pediatric patients is well defined. These children have relatively normal growth parameters until the age of 9 or 10 years, when growth velocity drops; onset of pubertal changes is delayed, and pubertal growth spurt is absent or very reduced; growth plate fusion happens in the their early twenties.[56] Studies on the use of GH therapy in children with beta-thalassemia are scant. GH treatment in 8 Chinese patients resulted in improved height standard deviation score after 3 years, with no deleterious effect on glucose metabolism seen in these children.[57] In a larger study, 283 prepubertal Sardinian children with beta-thalassemia major and GH deficiency were treated with GH for an average period of 59 months. Growth velocities in these patients normalized during the first year of therapy and remained within normal limits while on therapy.[49] No studies exist on the long-term use of GH therapy in this population.

GH Therapy in Chronic Kidney Disease

Chronic Kidney Disease (CKD) was the second indication overall and the first indication for a non-GH deficiency state approved by the FDA. CKD was approved as an indication in 1993, largely based on data from a multicenter trial.[58] Growth failure is significant for children with CKD, with as many as 35% of these patients affected.[59] The cause of this growth failure appears to be multifactorial. In part it is likely nutritional, related to the anorexia, nausea, and vomiting associated with uremic toxicity.[60] Additional factors include metabolic acidosis and renal osteodystrophy, and chronic inflammation may also play a role.[60] In addition, CKD causes disruption in the GH/IGF axis, including decreased expression of GH receptors, impairment of GH receptor transduction, decreased production of IGF-I, and decreased activity of IGF because of accumulation of inhibitory IGF binding proteins.[61–63] The involvement of the GH/IGF axis in the growth failure associated with CKD suggests that GH therapy may reverse some of the growth issues. Mahan and colleagues[64] examined the first-year growth velocity response to GH in children with CKD followed in the National Cooperative Growth Study (NCGS), and have shown that GH therapy results in a significant increase in growth velocity during the first year of treatment. An analysis of 16 studies has confirmed that GH therapy increases first-year growth velocity.[65] Second-year growth velocity was reduced, but remained significantly greater than in children with CKD not treated with GH. Notably, in addition to promoting linear growth in children with CKD, there is evidence that GH promotes an anabolic state, as demonstrated by increased body weight and midarm circumference measurements,[66] and it may also improve bone metabolism, resulting in improved bone mineral content and density.[67] All in all, in addition to increasing growth velocity in children with CKD, GH has been shown to increase serum IGF-I levels, lean body mass, bone turnover, and phagocytic activity of polymorphonuclear leukocytes, as well as decreasing body fat mass.[60]

The intent of the FDA indication was to offer GH to children with CKD until they received a kidney transplant. Unfortunately, after renal transplantation, growth failure remains an issue, due in part to graft dysfunction and corticosteroid administration for immunosuppressive therapy. Initially there was concern that GH might increase the risk of rejection of the graft, which was not actually borne out by early studies.[68] GH therapy increases the growth velocity of post-transplant patients,[68] and a series of 3 patients receiving GH after transplant suggests that GH therapy may increase final heights.[69]

Safety of GH

GH adverse events have been carefully documented in a review of GH therapy.[70] Most adverse events have been local injection site reactions, which rarely lead to discontinuation. Headache, nausea, and fever have been generally self-limiting and are well tolerated. Adverse events such as edema or carpal tunnel syndrome are seen more often in adults than children, and may be the result of fluid retention caused by GH.[71] Adverse events seen particularly in children have included transient idiopathic intracranial hypertension (IIH, also known as pseudotumor cerebri), gynecomastia, and slipped capital femoral epiphysis.[72,73] The IIH resolved after discontinuation of GH and restarting at a low dose.

Adverse events reported when GH is used in CKD include minor complaints, such as mild headaches, arthralgia, edema, nausea and vomiting, and paresthesia.[74] There have been a few more serious reports, including congestive heart failure and skin malignancies. Not observed were increases in rates of diabetes, left ventricular hypertrophy, or hypertension.

There have been concerns about cancer associated with GH administration. Acromegaly is known to increase the risk of colorectal cancer.[75] Epidemiologic studies have shown a relationship between tall statue and cancer risk,[76] between IGF-I levels and the risk of prostate cancer,[77] and an increase in breast cancer associated with levels of free IGF-I.[78] One study[79] has suggested that there may be reason for concern because of cases of Hodgkin disease and colorectal cancer found in long-term follow-up of patients who had received human-derived GH. Although the incidence of these diseases was greater than the population at large, it was not outside the confidence ranges. Further, follow-up of patients receiving human-derived GH in the United States[79] has not shown such a correlation. There has been recent concern from analysis of data in French children who were treated with GH between 1985 and 1996, and then followed until 1996 (the Safety and Appropriateness of GH use in Europe (SAGhE) study).[80] A retrospective analysis of mortality in this population suggests the possibility of increased cardiovascular disease and bone tumors in adults who received GH as children. The cardiovascular disease was primarily attributed to subarachnoid or intracerebral hemorrhages. Overall cancer mortality rates were not higher than the general population, but bone tumor-related deaths were 5 times higher than expected. There appeared to be a dose relationship (risk was highest in patients receiving doses >50 μg/d). However, there was no apparent relationship with duration of GH therapy, which one would expect if the increase in mortality was actually related to GH therapy. Data from other European countries should be available over the next several years, and may shed some light on the SAGhE data. A recent report[81] examines life expectancy in 99 Ecuadorian people with GH receptor deficiency (GHRD), that is, who had a defect in their GH receptor, leading to IGF-I deficiency. The GHRD population had only 1 cancer (not fatal), compared with 17% of the control population. Further, there were no cases of diabetes in the GHRD population, compared with 5% in the control population. This study provides strong evidence that the GHRD population has resistance to cancer and diabetes.

Overall, GH has been shown to be a safe hormone when used at recommended doses. There are excellent large databases for evaluation of possible safety signals that occur during treatment with GH. What is most needed is long-term adult follow-up of those patients who received GH as children.

SUMMARY

From careful studies over the past 25 years, GH appears to be a relatively safe hormone, at least during the time that it is being administered. There are few data relating to long-term follow-up, and this is a challenge for the future. GH is a powerful growth-promoting anabolic hormone, which may have further use in treating a number of short stature conditions, for example Russell-Silver syndrome or chondrodystrophies, as well as X-linked vitamin D-resistant rickets. When used to treat CF, it may offer stimulation of linear growth, as well as better energy balance. Height- and non-height0related benefits of GH therapy in patients suffering from chronic inflammatory conditions like JIA and CD have been demonstrated and will need to be further studied. The steroid-sparing effect of GH therapy appears promising in many of these conditions. Strictly controlled trials of GH use in burn patients, beta-thalassemia, and rickets are needed in the future, as preliminary results have been positive. GH should not be used in critically ill patients, since it has been associated with increased mortality in this population. It may possibly offer benefit to situations of muscle wasting, including aging, and it does appear to offer some advantage in physical performance, which may lead to uses in treating injured patients who could benefit from increased physical function and independence. Further studies are indicated to determine the risks and benefits, as well as the cost relative to the benefits for a number of conditions.

REFERENCES

1. Raben MS. Treatment of a pituitary dwarf with human growth hormone. J Clin Endocrinol Metab 1958;18:901.
2. Hardin DS. GH improves growth and clinical status in children with cystic fibrosis—a review of published studies. Eur J Endocrinol 2004;151:s81.
3. Hardin DS, Ellis K, Dyson M, et al. Growth hormone improves clinical status in children with cystic fibrosis—results of a randomized controlled trial. J Pediatr 2001;139:636.
4. Hardin DS, Rice J, Ahn C, et al. Growth hormone treatment enhances nutrition and growth in children with cystic fibrosis receiving enteral nutrition. J Pediatr 2005;146:324.
5. Phung OJ, Coleman CI, Baker EL, et al. Recombinant human growth hormone in the treatment of patients with cystic fibrosis. Pediatrics 2010;126:e1211.
6. Stalvey MS, Anbar RD, Konstan MV, et al. A multi-center controlled trial of growth hormone treatment in children with cystic fibrosis. Pediatr Pulmonol 2012;47:252.
7. MacRae VE, Wong SC, Farquharson C, et al. Cytokine actions in growth disorders associated with pediatric chronic inflammatory diseases (review). Int J Mol Med 2006;18:1011.
8. Zak M, Muller J, Karup Pedersen F. Final height, armspan, subischial leg length and body proportions in juvenile chronic arthritis. A long-term follow-up study. Horm Res 1999;52:80.
9. Simon D, Lucidarme N, Prieur AM, et al. Treatment of growth failure in juvenile chronic arthritis. Horm Res 2002;1(Suppl 58):28.
10. Wang SJ, Yang YH, Lin YT, et al. Attained adult height in juvenile rheumatoid arthritis with or without corticosteroid treatment. Clin Rheumatol 2002;21:363.
11. De Benedetti F, Meazza C, Oliveri M, et al. Effect of IL-6 on IGF binding protein-3: a study in IL-6 transgenic mice and in patients with systemic juvenile idiopathic arthritis. Endocrinology 2001;142:4818.
12. Davies UM, Jones J, Reeve J, et al. Juvenile rheumatoid arthritis. Effects of disease activity and recombinant human growth hormone on insulin-like growth factor 1, insulin-like growth factor binding proteins 1 and 3, and osteocalcin. Arthritis Rheum 1997;40:332.
13. Tsatsoulis A, Siamopoulou A, Petsoukis C, et al. Study of growth hormone secretion and action in growth-retarded children with juvenile chronic arthritis (JCA). Growth Horm IGF Res 1999;9:143.
14. Lazarus DD, Moldawer LL, Lowry SF. Insulin-like growth factor-1 activity is inhibited by interleukin-1 alpha, tumor necrosis factor-alpha, and interleukin-6. Lymphokine Cytokine Res 1993;12:219.
15. Gaspari S, Marcovecchio ML, Breda L, et al. Growth in juvenile idiopathic arthritis: the role of inflammation. Clin Exp Rheumatol 2011;29:104.
16. Simon D, Bechtold S. Effects of growth hormone treatment on growth in children with juvenile idiopathic arthritis. Horm Res 2009;1(Suppl 72):55.
17. Bechtold S, Ripperger P, Dalla Pozza R, et al. Dynamics of body composition and bone in patients with juvenile idiopathic arthritis treated with growth hormone. J Clin Endocrinol Metab 2010;95:178.
18. Sawczenko A, Ballinger AB, Croft NM, et al. Adult height in patients with early onset of Crohn's disease. Gut 2003;52:454.

19. Denson LA, Kim MO, Bezold R, et al. A randomized controlled trial of growth hormone in active pediatric Crohn disease. J Pediatr Gastroenterol Nutr 2010; 51:130.

20. Slonim AE, Bulone L, Damore MB, et al. A preliminary study of growth hormone therapy for Crohn's disease. N Engl J Med 2000;342:1633.

21. Mauras N, George D, Evans J, et al. Growth hormone has anabolic effects in glucocorticosteroid-dependent children with inflammatory bowel disease: a pilot study. Metabolism 2002;51:127.

22. Heyman MB, Garnett EA, Wojcicki J, et al. Growth hormone treatment for growth failure in pediatric patients with crohn's disease. J Pediatr 2008;153:651.

23. Schakman O, Gilson H, Thissen JP. Mechanisms of glucocorticoid-induced myopathy. J Endocrinol 2008;197:1.

24. Hardin DS, Adams-Huet B, Brown D, et al. Growth hormone treatment improves growth and clinical status in prepubertal children with cystic fibrosis: results of a multicenter randomized controlled trial. J Clin Endocrinol Metab 2006;91:4925.

25. Darmaun D, Hayes V, Schaeffer D, et al. Effects of glutamine and recombinant human growth hormone on protein metabolism in prepubertal children with cystic fibrosis. J Clin Endocrinol Metab 2004;89:1146.

26. Ruokonen E, Takala J. Dangers of growth hormone therapy in critically ill patients. Curr Opin Clin Nutr Metab Care 2002;5:199.

27. Takala J, Ruokonen E, Webster NR, et al. Increased mortality associated with growth hormone treatment in critically ill adults. N Engl J Med 1999;341:785.

28. Herndon DN, Barrow RE, Kunkel KR, et al. Effects of recombinant human growth hormone on donor-site healing in severely burned children. Ann Surg 1990;212: 430.

29. Lal SO, Wolf SE, Herndon DN. Growth hormone, burns and tissue healing. Growth Horm IGF Res 2000;10:S39.

30. Hart DW, Herndon DN, Klein G, et al. Attenuation of posttraumatic muscle catabolism and osteopenia by long-term growth hormone therapy. Ann Surg 2001;233: 827.

31. Gore DC, Honeycutt D, Jahoor F, et al. Effect of exogenous growth hormone on whole-body and isolated-limb protein kinetics in burned patients. Arch Surg 1991;126:38.

32. Herndon DN, Pierre EJ, Stokes KN, et al. Growth hormone treatment for burned children. Horm Res 1996;1(Suppl 45):29.

33. Herndon DN, Hawkins HK, Nguyen TT, et al. Characterization of growth hormone enhanced donor site healing in patients with large cutaneous burns. Ann Surg 1995;221:649.

34. Takagi K, Suzuki F, Barrow RE, et al. Recombinant human growth hormone modulates Th1 and Th2 cytokine response in burned mice. Ann Surg 1998;228:106.

35. Low JF, Herndon DN, Barrow RE. Effect of growth hormone on growth delay in burned children: a 3-year follow-up study. Lancet 1999;354:1789.

36. Jeschke MG, Finnerty CC, Kulp GA, et al. Combination of recombinant human growth hormone and propranolol decreases hypermetabolism and inflammation in severely burned children. Pediatr Crit Care Med 2008;9:209.

37. Branski LK, Herndon DN, Barrow RE, et al. Randomized controlled trial to determine the efficacy of long-term growth hormone treatment in severely burned children. Ann Surg 2009;250:514.

38. Delehaye-Zervas MC, Mertani H, Martini JF, et al. Expression of the growth hormone receptor gene in human digestive tissue. J Clin Endocrinol Metab 1994;78:1473.

39. Byrne TA, Persinger RL, Young LS, et al. A new treatment for patients with short-bowel syndrome. Growth hormone, glutamine, and a modified diet. Ann Surg 1995;222:243.

40. Scolapio JS. Effect of growth hormone, glutamine, and diet on body composition in short bowel syndrome: a randomized, controlled study. JPEN J Parenter Enteral Nutr 1999;23:309.

41. Velasco B, Lassaletta L, Gracia R, et al. Intestinal lengthening and growth hormone in extreme short bowel syndrome: a case report. J Pediatr Surg 1999; 34:1423.

42. McMellen ME, Wakeman D, Longshore SW, et al. Growth factors: possible roles for clinical management of the short bowel syndrome. Semin Pediatr Surg 2010; 19:35.

43. Saggese G, Baroncelli GI, Barsanti S. Growth hormone treatment of familial hypophosphatemic rickets. Arch Pediatr 1998;5:360S.

44. Saggese G, Baroncelli GI, Bartellone S, et al. Long-term growth hormone treatment in children with renal hypophosphatemic rickets: effect on growth mineral metabolism, and bone density. J Pediatr 1995;127:395.

45. Reusz GS, Miltényi G, Stubnya G, et al. X-linked hypophosphatemia: effects of treatment with recombinant human growth hormone. Pediatr Nephrol 1997;11: 573.

46. Wilson DM. Growth hormone and hypophosphatemic rickets. J Pediatr Endocrinol Metab 2000;13:993.

47. Baroncelli GI, Bertelloni S, Ceccarelli C, et al. Effect of growth hormone treatment on final height, phosphate metabolism, and bone mineral density in children with X-linked hypophosphatemic rickets. J Pediatr 2001;138:236–43.

48. Huiming Y, Chaomin W. Recombinant growth hormone therapy for X-linked hypophosphatemia in children. Cochrane Database Syst Rev 2005;(1):CD004447.

49. Masala A, Atzeni MM, Alagna S, et al. Growth hormone secretion in polytransfused prepubertal patients with homozygous beta-thalassemia. Effect of long-term recombinant GH (recGH) therapy. J Endocrinol Invest 2003;26:623.

50. Wu KH, Tsai FJ, Peng CT. Growth hormone (GH) deficiency in patients with beta-thalassemia major and the efficacy of recombinant GH treatment. Ann Hematol 2003;82:637.

51. Erfurth EM, Holmer H, Nilsson PG, et al. Is growth hormone deficiency contributing to heart failure in patients with beta-thalassemia major? Eur J Endocrinol 2004;151:161.

52. Karydis I, Karagiorga-Lagana M, Nounopoulos C, et al. Basal and stimulated levels of growth hormone, insulin-like growth factor-I (IGF-I), IGF-I binding and IGF-binding proteins in beta-thalassemia major. J Pediatr Endocrinol Metab 2004;17:17.

53. Moayeri H, Oloomi Z. Prevalence of growth and puberty failure with respect to growth hormone and gonadotropins secretion in beta-thalassemia major. Arch Iran Med 2006;9:329.

54. Vidergor G, Goldfarb AW, Glaser B, et al. Growth hormone reserve in adult beta thalassemia patients. Endocrine 2007;31:33.

55. Poggi M, Pascucci C, Monti S, et al. Prevalence of growth hormone deficiency in adult polytransfused beta-thalassemia patients and correlation with transfusional and chelation parameters. J Endocrinol Invest 2010;33:534.

56. Rodda CP, Reid ED, Johnson S, et al. Short stature in homozygous beta-thalassaemia is due to disproportionate truncal shortening. Clin Endocrinol (Oxf) 1995;42:587.

57. Kwan EY, Tam SC, Cheung PT, et al. The effect of 3 years of recombinant growth hormone therapy on glucose metabolism in short Chinese children with beta-thalassemia major. J Pediatr Endocrinol Metab 2000;13:545.

58. Fine RN, Kohaut EC, Brown D, et al. Growth after recombinant growth hormone treatment in children with chronic renal failure: report of a multicenter randomized double-blind placebo-controlled study. Genentech cooperative study group. J Pediatr 1994;124:374.

59. Seikaly MG, Salhab N, Warady BA, et al. Use of rhGH in children with chronic kidney disease. Lessons from NAPRTCS. Pediatr Nephrol 2007;22:1195.

60. Gupta V, Lee M. Growth hormone in chronic renal disease. Indian J Endocrinol Metab 2012;16:195.

61. Rabkin R, Sun DF, Chen Y, et al. Growth hormone resistance in uremia, a role for impaired JAK/STAT signaling. Pediatr Nephrol 2005;20:313.

62. Roelfsema V, Clark RG. The growth hormone and insulin-like growth factor axis: its manipulation for the benefit of growth disorders in renal failure. J Am Soc Nephrol 2001;12:1297.

63. Tonshoff B, Kiepe D, Ciarmatori S. Growth hormone/insulin-like growth factor system in children with chronic renal failure. Pediatr Nephrol 2005;20:279.

64. Mahan JD, Warady BA, Frane J, et al. First-year response to rhGH therapy in children with CKD: a national cooperative growth study report. Pediatr Nephrol 2010; 25:1125.

65. Hodson EM, Willis NS, Craig JC. Growth hormone for children wtih chronic kidney disease. Cochrane Database Syst Rev 2012;(2):CD003264.

66. Fine RN, Yadin O, Moulton L, et al. Five years experience with recombinant human growth hormone treatment of children with chronic renal failure. J Pediatr Endocrinol 1994;7:1.

67. Van Dyck M, Gyssels A, Proesmans W, et al. Growth hormone treatment enhances bone mineralisation in children with chronic renal failure. Eur J Pediatr 2001;160:359.

68. Mentser M, Breen TJ, Sullivan EK, et al. Growth-hormone treatment of renal transplant recipients: the National Cooperative Growth Study experience—a report of the National Cooperative Growth Study and the North American Pediatric Renal Transplant Cooperative Study. J Pediatr 1997;131:S20.

69. Motoyama O, Hasegawa A, Kawamura T, et al. Adult height of three renal transplant patients after growth hormone therapy. Clin Exp Nephrol 2007;11: 332.

70. Krysiak R, Gdula-Dymek A, Bednarska-Czerwińska A, et al. Growth hormone therapy in children and adults. Pharmacol Rep 2007;59:500.

71. Cummings DE, Merriam GR. Growth hormone therapy in adults. Annu Rev Med 2003;54:513.

72. Festen DA, van Toorenenbergen A, Duivenvoorden HJ, et al. Adiponectin level in prepubertal children with prader-willi syndrome before and after growth hormone therapy. J Clin Endocrinol Metab 2007;90:5156.

73. Root AW, Root MJ. Clinical pharmacology of human growth hormone and its secretagogues. Curr Drug Targets Immune Endocr Metabol Disord 2002;2:27.

74. Gupta D, Gardner M, Whaley-Connell A. Role of growth hormone deficiency and treatment in chronic kidney disease. Cardiorenal Med 2011;1:174.

75. Renehan AG, Brennan BM. Acromegaly, growth hormone and cancer risk. Best Pract Res Clin Endocrinol Metab 2008;22:639.

76. Gunnell D, Okasha M, Smith GD, et al. Height, leg length, and cancer risk: a systematic review. Epidemiol Rev 2008;23:313.

77. Rowlands MA, Gunnell D, Harris R, et al. Circulating insulin-like growth factor peptides and prostate cancer risk: a systematic review and meta-analysis. Int J Cancer 2009;124:2416.

78. Peyrat JP, Bonneterre J, Hecquet B, et al. Plasma insulin-like growth factor-1 (IGF-1) concentrations in human breast cancer. Eur J Cancer 1993;29A:492.

79. Swerdlow AJ, Higgins CD, Adlard P, et al. Risk of cancer in patients treated with human pituitary growth hormone in the UK, 1959–85: a cohort study. Lancet 2002; 360:273.

80. Carel J-C, Ecosse E, Landier F, et al. Long-term mortality after recombinant growth hormone treatment for isolated growth hormone deficiency or childhood short stature: Preliminary report of the French SAGhE study. J Clin Endocrinol Metab 2012;97:416.

81. Guevara-Aguirre J. Growth hormone receptor deficiency is associated with a major reduction in pro-aging signaling, cancer, and diabetes in humans. Sci Transl Med 2011;3:70ra13.

A Pathophysiologic Approach to Growth Problems in Children with Attention-Deficit/Hyperactivity Disorder

Alfred Tenore, MD[a,b,*], Andrew Tenore, MD[a]

KEYWORDS

- Attention-deficit/hyperactivity disorder • Sleep • Growth • Neurotransmitters
- Central nervous system • Weight • Puberty

KEY POINTS

- Currently 2 main criteria are in use for the diagnosis of attention-deficit/hyperactivity disorder (ADHD): (1) the *International Classification of Mental and Behavioral Disorders, Tenth Revision* and (2) the *Diagnostic and Statistical Manual of Mental Disorders, Fourth Edition*.
- The 6 main brain (cognitive) functions that seem to be affected in individuals with ADHD[1] are activation, focus, effort, memory, action, and emotion.

INTRODUCTION

Most children with attention-deficit/hyperactivity disorder (ADHD) benefit from taking specific medication, which, although it does not cure the disorder, can make a big difference in improving their ability to pay attention and control their behavior so that they can function at a normal level and focus while in school. However, just like any other medication, drugs used for ADHD can have side effects. One of the most talked about and controversial effects of these medications is on linear growth.

In order to understand (it would be presumptuous to use "clarify") the problem of growth in ADHD, it is important to review some of the important information currently available on this disorder. Therefore, this article, in discussing this controversial problem, analyzes, as best as possible, what ADHD is both from a clinical and from a biochemical perspective, its pathogenesis, and what intrinsic characteristics of

[a] Division of Pediatric Endocrinology, Department of Pediatrics, DSMSC, University of Udine, Udine 33100, Italy; [b] European Academy of Paediatrics - Paediatric Section of UEMS, Brussels, Belgium
* Corresponding author. Via Gemona 52/A, Udine 33100, Italy.
E-mail address: altenusa@gmail.com

Endocrinol Metab Clin N Am 41 (2012) 761–784
http://dx.doi.org/10.1016/j.ecl.2012.08.004

the disorder may be associated with the normal process of growth. The article also looks at the basic neurophysiologic mechanisms involved in growth hormone (GH) secretion and relates how these could be disrupted by the underlying mechanisms presumed responsible for ADHD or its medical stimulant treatment.

WHAT IS ADHD?

Contrary to popular belief, the first example of a disorder that seems to be similar to ADHD was given a little more than 200 years ago in 1798 by Sir Alexander Crichton (1763–1856), a Scottish physician, with the publication of a 3-volume book in which his description of the first alteration of attention gives several indications that he was describing the same disorder as defined by the criteria for ADHD in the current, text-revised edition of the *Diagnostic and Statistical Manual of Mental Disorders, Fourth Edition* (DSM-IV-TR).[2] In 1845, Dr Heinrich Hoffman, a German physician considered to be the first representative of child and adolescent psychiatry, wrote a book of poems (later known as *Struwwelpeter*) about children and their personalities. In one of these poems, entitled *The Story of Fidgety Philip*, Dr Hoffman gives an accurate description of a child with ADHD.[3] In 1902, Sir George F. Still, England's first professor of child medicine, provided the first clinical description of the disorder in a series of lectures to the Royal College of Physicians in London, under the title "Goulstonian lectures on 'Some abnormal psychical conditions in children'", which were published later the same year in *The Lancet*.[4] Still described 43 children who displayed impulsivity and behavior problems. According to Still, these symptoms were caused by a genetic dysfunction and not by poor parenting. In 1937 appeared the first report using a stimulant medication (benzedrine) to treat hyperactivity.[5] Methylphenidate, which is still considered the drug of first choice, was synthesized in 1944 by Leandro Panizzon and marketed as Ritalin by Ciba-Geigy Pharmaceutical Company in 1954. The name Ritalin derives from the first name of Panizzon's wife (Marguerite or Rita).

Before acquiring the current name of ADHD, this entity went through a variety of other names, such as postencephalitic behavior disorder after the worldwide spread of epidemics of encephalitis between 1917 and 1928, hyperkinetic disorder (~1930s), minimal brain damage (~1940–1960s), minimal brain dysfunction (MBD)[6] (~1960–1980s). The idea of a hyperkinetic impulse disorder was continued in the 1960s, and the concept of a hyperactivity syndrome was generated. In 1968, DSM-II recognized the label hyperkinetic reaction of childhood. In the 1970s, the predominant focus on hyperactivity was shifted towards an emphasis on attention deficit in affected children. In 1980, the importance of attention problems in the syndrome was recognized, and with the publication of DSM-III in 1980, the American Psychiatric Association renamed the disorder attention-deficit disorder (ADD) (with or without hyperactivity). In this respect, DSM-III departed from the *International Classification of Diseases* (ICD-9) by the World Health Organization, which continued to focus on hyperactivity as an indicator of the disorder. However, with DSM-IV, the disorder was renamed attention-deficit/hyperactivity disorder.

ADHD or hyperkinetic disorder, as referred to by the World Health Organization and defined by ICD-10,[7] is one of the most common health disorders in children. Polanczyk and colleagues,[8] in a systematic review and metaregression analysis of the global prevalence of ADHD, found that the worldwide pooled prevalence is 5.3%, with highly variable rates ranging from 1% to almost 20% among school-aged children. Furthermore, the study also found that no significant differences were detected in the prevalence between North America and Europe, although several investigators had previously suggested that ADHD was primarily an American condition[9] or a cultural construct.[10]

The American Psychiatric Association defines ADHD as "a syndrome whose hallmarks are inattention" (a disorganized style preventing sustained effort), "hyperactivity" (restless and shifting excess of movement), and "impulsivity" (premature and thoughtless actions), the symptoms of which "are expressed in multiple settings and across numerous functional domains, thus demonstrating the pervasiveness of this condition."[11] However, not all individuals with ADHD have all 3 symptoms, and although these 3 symptoms cluster together, some individuals are primarily inattentive, whereas others are hyperactive and impulsive. In boys, in whom ADHD is more commonly found than in girls, the male/female ratio for the predominantly inattentive type is 2:1, whereas for the predominantly hyperactive type it is 4:1.[12,13] In general, ADHD is a persistent disorder because most of the children/adolescents with a sustained diagnosis have significant difficulties as adults, such as persistent ADHD, emotional/social difficulties, personality disorders, substance misuse/abuse, unemployment, and unlawful actions.

Cross-cultural research has shown that ADHD exists in all cultures, with increased access to public education being a factor in its detection. In line with this statement is a study that was conducted in the Washington, DC metropolitan area. Information was obtained through an anonymous survey sent to primary care pediatricians, family physicians, and child psychiatrists asking who first suggests the diagnosis of ADHD. The results indicated that teachers along with other school personnel accounted for 52% of the identifications and parents for 30%, as opposed to primary care physicians, who accounted for only 11%.[14] However, although school personnel are theoretically more dependable in picking out the fidgety and inattentive child, there is still some concern regarding the teacher's accuracy in suggesting such a diagnosis.

Currently, 2 main criteria are in use for the diagnosis of ADHD: ICD-10 and DSM-IV. The basic difference between the 2 is that ICD-10 uses a narrower diagnostic category, including individuals with more severe symptoms and impairment, whereas DSM-IV has a broader, more inclusive definition and thus includes several different ADHD subtypes (the prevalence of ADHD may vary depending on which diagnostic criteria are used). **Box 1** includes the criteria used in DSM-IV, which serve as a guideline for determining the presence of ADHD. However, it is recommended that a diagnosis of ADHD be made only by a specialist psychiatrist, pediatrician, or other qualified health care professional with training and expertise in diagnosing ADHD.[15] Essential to making a diagnosis of ADHD is that the characteristic symptoms of hyperactivity, impulsivity, or inattention should (1) meet the criteria in DSM-IV or ICD-10, (2) be associated with at least moderate psychological, social, and educational impairment based on direct observation in multiple settings, and (3) occur in 2 or more settings (ie, social, familial, or educational).

Because mental disorders such as depression and anxiety can cause symptoms similar to ADHD, it is important to follow such guidelines for proper diagnosis so that such disorders do not receive inappropriate stimulant treatment. Some investigators have questioned whether all children receiving medication for ADHD meet standard diagnostic criteria for ADHD,[16] which in part could be the reason why the use of ADHD medications has been steadily increasing worldwide. Scheffler and colleagues[17] reported an increased use of such medications of 274% over an 11-year period between 1993 and 2003, with a steady increase of 13.2% per year from 1993 to 2000 and 16.8% per year from 2000 to 2003. This trend has continued to show a steady increase based on the most recent data by Chai and colleagues,[18] who looked at trends of outpatient prescription drug use in the United States between 2002 and 2010 and found that whereas the use of systemic antibiotics decreased by 14%, the use of ADHD drugs increased by 46%, representing the largest increasing trend of all prescribed medications (0.8 million prescriptions/y). Given the global

---

Box 1
DSM-IV Diagnostic Criteria for the Diagnosis of ADHD

For a diagnosis of ADHD, DSM-IV requires the presence of at least 6 of the symptoms listed under "inattention," or 6 or more symptoms of those listed under "hyperactivity" and "impulsivity" combined and have persisted for at least 6 months to a degree that is not "maladptive and inconsistent with developmental level."

Inattention

- avoids or dislikes tasks that require sustained mental effort (eg, homework)
- does not seem to listen when spoken to
- does not follow through on instructions and does not finish tasks
- fails to pay close attention to detail or makes careless mistakes in schoolwork or other activities
- has difficulty organizing tasks and activities
- has difficulty sustaining attention in tasks or activities
- is easily distracted
- is forgetful in daily activities

Hyperactivity

- does not remain seated when expected to
- fidgets with hands or feet or squirms in seat
- has difficulty playing quietly
- is constantly on the move
- runs or climbs excessively when inappropriate (in adolescents and adults, feelings of restlessness)
- talks excessively

Impulsivity

- blunts out answers before the question has been completed
- has difficulty waiting for their turn
- interrupts or intrudes on others

Adapted from American Psychiatric Association. Diagnostic and statistical manual of mental disorders (DSM-4). 4th edition. Washington, DC: American Psychiatric Press; 2000.

---

diffusion of ADHD medications, as well as the prevalence of this condition, ADHD could, if it has not already, become the leading childhood disorder treated with medications across the globe.

CAUSES OF ADHD

The cause (or causes) for the development of ADHD continue to be unclear, even although there is strong evidence, and it is generally accepted, that ADHD involves the interplay of multiple genetic and environmental factors. The genetic evidence comes from studies involving twins and adopted children with ADHD as well as studies looking at the rates of occurrence of ADHD within families. From the numerous twin studies that have been performed from various parts of the world in the last 30 years, the average concordance rate found was 76% in monozygotic twins[19] and 33% in same-sexed dizygotic twins.[20] Adoption studies found that the percentage of parents who were retrospectively hyperactive as children were 18% in the biologic parents versus 6% in the adopting parents, and 3% in the biological parents of the control group.[21] With regard to family studies, 30% to 35% of full siblings of affected children also met ADHD criteria,[22] and ADHD was present in more than 25% of first-degree relatives of families having children with ADHD.[23] Although genetic studies unequivocally indicate that genes are risk factors for this disorder, they also show that environmental determinants have a strong influence on the development of the disorder. The fact that identical twins have only about a 70% concordance rate implicates a significant influence of environmental risk factors at work.

However, regardless of the numerous multidisciplinary studies that have been conducted over the years, it seems clear that there is still no single cause to explain ADHD, possibly because ADHD does not represent a single entity. As pointed out earlier, ADHD is characterized by the 3 classic symptoms of inattention, hyperactivity, and impulsivity, which, although they cluster together, may appear in various combinations. For this reason, DSM-IV recognizes 3 subtypes: (1) the predominantly hyperactive-impulsive type (who do not show significant inattention); (2) the predominantly inattentive type (who do not show significant hyperactive-impulsive behavior) and (3) the combined type (who show both inattentive and hyperactive-impulsive symptoms) (**Box 2**). Because inattention, hyperactivity, and impulsivity are controlled in different areas of the central nervous system (CNS), it could imply that selective areas of the CNS may be involved depending on the predominant clinical expression. Therefore, the search for a unifying cause of ADHD may be hampered by the heterogeneity of the disorder.

ADHD is increasingly being recognized as a disorder affecting executive functions (EF) (ie, a wide range of central cognitive functions that play a critical role in the management of multiple tasks of daily life). The 6 main brain (cognitive) functions that seem to be affected in individuals with ADHD[1] are:

1. Activation (difficulty in organization of thoughts, ideas, and getting started on a task)
2. Focus (difficulty in sustaining interest, changing from 1 topic/idea to another)
3. Effort (difficulty regulating alertness and sleep and maintaining effort in the completion of tasks over prolonged periods and on time)
4. Memory (difficulty in taking in, storing, and retrieving information effectively)
5. Action (difficulty in acting appropriately for lack of adequate consideration of the consequences)
6. Emotion (difficulty in managing frustration, anger, disappointments, and other emotions)

Although the control of emotion is not part of the DSM-IV criteria for the diagnosis of ADHD, many patients have difficulty in their control.[24]

Box 2
There are 3 types of ADHD. Some children with ADHD show symptoms of inattention and are not hyperactive or impulsive. Others show only symptoms of hyperactivity-impulsivity. However, most show symptoms of both inattention and hyperactivity-impulsivity

- Predominantly inattentive type
- Predominantly hyperactive-impulsive type
- Combined type

The altered functions described in patients with ADHD suggest that several areas of the brain may be affected by this disorder. Functional neurophysiologic-imaging studies[25–28] are consistent with structural studies[29] in locating abnormalities of brain activation in individuals with ADHD to the frontosubcortical-cerebellar circuits,[30] as well as showing a reduction in gray matter in the right putamen/globus pallidus region (lenticular nucleus).[31] Taken collectively, the most recent models describing what is happening neurologically in the brains of individuals with ADHD suggest the involvement of several areas of the brain. These areas include (1) the frontal lobe, important for the EF of focus, action and memory, (2) the cortex (ie, the inhibitory mechanism of the cortex), important for controlling hyperactivity and impulsiveness; when the inhibitory mechanisms of the cortex are not working appropriately it results in disinhibition disorders such as hyperactivity, impulsive behaviors, quick temper, and poor decision-making, and (3) the limbic system (LS) (ie, hypothalamus, a collection of interconnected structures in the telencephalon, as well as the amygdale and hippocampal formation). A normally functioning LS provides for normal emotional changes, levels of energy, sleep routines, and ability to cope with stress. ADHD might affect these areas singly or in any combination, resulting in different clinical manifestations of the disorder.

A fourth area of the brain that also seems to be affected is the reticular activating system (RAS), which is composed of the reticular formation in the midbrain, the mesencephalic nucleus, and portions of the thalamus and hypothalamus. This system is represented by a complex collection of neurons that serve as a point of convergence for signals between the external and internal environments. It represents the center of balance for the other systems involved in motivation, learning, and self-control or inhibition. When functioning normally, it provides the neural connections that are needed for the processing and learning of information, and the ability to pay attention to the correct task. If the RAS does not excite the neurons of the cortex appropriately, what should result is an underaroused cortex. In line with this premise are research findings that show that most children with ADHD, when compared with normal children, have electroencephalograms that are associated most consistently with increased θ activity, indicating that cortical underarousal is a common neuropathologic mechanism in ADHD.[32]

The RAS is also intimately involved in the neural mechanisms that produce consciousness and focused attention, receiving impulses from the spinal cord, relaying them to the thalamus, then to the cortex and back, in a feedback loop, to the hippocampus/thalamus/hypothalamus and the participating neural structure in order for learning and memory to take place. Neuropsychological studies have suggested that the frontal cortex and the circuits that link them to the basal ganglia are critical for the execution of EF and that catecholamines are the main neurotransmitters in the circuits involved in frontal-lobe functions (**Fig. 1**). In addition, attention and vigilance also depend on adequate modulation by catecholamine neurotransmitters of prefrontal, cingulate and parietal cortices, thalamus, striatum, and hippocampus, all areas that have a high density of catecholamine terminals. Therefore, it is not by chance that the use of medications that are directed towards the catecholamine control of dopaminergic and noradrenergic neurotransmission have been and continue to be the mainstay of treatment of ADHD. Many review articles assert that ADHD is caused by a deficit of the catecholaminergic system, the origin of which is considered to be primarily genetic.

Recent studies confirm previous hypotheses concerning the role of genetic variation within genes that are involved in the regulation of catecholamine neurotransmitters in ADHD.[33,34] However, despite the identification of several candidate genes, none of them seems to have a substantial effect in the contribution to ADHD.

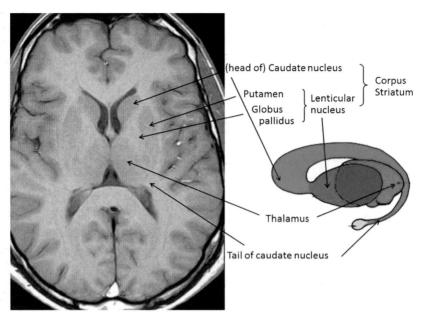

Fig. 1. Basal ganglia (nucleus). The right side of the figure depicts the components of the corpus striatum with their corresponding projections on a transverse section of a magnetic resonance imaging scan of the brain. Findings from neurophysiologic studies suggest that the frontal cortex and the circuits linking them to the basal ganglia are critical for EF in ADHD.

Nevertheless, considering the enormous amount of information that has accumulated on this subject over the years, there is considerable evidence from animal and human studies to implicate the dysregulation of frontal-subcortical-cerebellar catecholaminergic circuits in the pathophysiology of ADHD, and molecular imaging studies suggest that abnormalities of the dopamine transporter (DAT) lead to impaired neurotransmission.

NEUROTRANSMITTERS

Intercellular communication in the CNS requires the precise control of the duration and the intensity of neurotransmitter action at specific molecular targets. There are 3 major categories of substances that act as neurotransmitters: (1) amino acids (primarily glutamic acid, γ-aminobutyric acid (GABA), aspartic acid, and glycine), (2) neuropeptides (eg, somatostatin (SS), vasopressin, neurotensin) and (3) monoamines. The primary monoamine neurotransmitters are dopamine, norepinephrine (both catecholamines) and serotonin (an indolamine). There are 3 to 4 times more dopaminergic cells in the CNS than adrenergic cells. Although there are more than 50 different neurotransmitters in the CNS, the peripheral nervous system has only 2, acetylcholine and norepinephrine.

A theory of adrenergic dysregulation has been proposed to explain ADHD, but studies that have investigated adrenergic metabolites in blood, platelets, and urine in children with ADHD, compared with normal children, have found contradictory results. One possible explanation for this finding may be that although concentrations of neurotransmitters in the brain range from micromolar to fentomolar quantities, the critical functional concentration of a neurotransmitter is that existing at the synapse. Because synaptic neurotransmitter levels are not measurable, it is not possible to clearly establish which concentration of any neurotransmitter is physiologic as opposed to pharmacologic. Furthermore, the behavioral effect of any specific neurotransmitter is highly dependent on the anatomic site at which it is released. Nevertheless, indirect support for what has come to be known as the catecholamine hypothesis to explain ADHD comes from several clinical and experimental observations, which include: (1) effective medical treatments seem to have an adrenergic mechanism of action in common; (2) studies in mouse[35] and monkey[36] models implicate dopaminergic pathways; (3) studies using the spontaneously hypertensive rat (an animal model of ADHD) show deficits in catecholaminergic systems[37]; (4) D2, D3, and D4 knockout mice studies[38,39] show that these genes regulate locomotor activity; and (5) rat[40,41] and human studies that implicate the DRD4[42] and DAT[43] genes in the genesis of ADHD.

Based on this evidence, it is safe to say, at least for the moment, that ADHD is associated with dysregulation of several neurotransmitter systems. A logical extension of this premise is that this dysregulation may alter neuroendocrine function and lead, among other things, to problems in growth that have been inconsistently reported in the literature. The physiologic mechanisms that underlie growth suppression remain obscure, in part because of our limited understanding of the pathophysiology of ADHD.

Two points emerge that are important for the discussion on growth: (1) most of the areas in the CNS that are involved in ADHD are also those responsible for the secretion of GH, and (2) the neurotransmitters that have been found to be altered in ADHD are the same as those responsible for GH secretion. The natural deduction from this type of reasoning could suggest that the child with ADHD may be at risk for growth problems regardless of whether they are being treated.

The next section discusses some of the factors that physiologically control GH secretion and relates them to what may be happening in the child with ADHD whether or not on treatment. In this regard, an important initial question needs to be answered: whether growth suppression (height and weight) is an intrinsic characteristic of ADHD.

GH SECRETION

The secretion of GH is regulated through a complex neuroendocrine control system consisting of multiple neurotransmitter pathways, as well as a variety of peripheral feedback signals, either by acting directly on the anterior pituitary gland or by modulating GH-releasing hormone (GHRH) or SS release, or both, from the hypothalamus. Current knowledge indicates that GH secretion depends on the interplay between GHRH and SS on the somatotrope. The secretion of both GHRH and SS is in turn controlled by a complex network of neurons through specific neurotransmitters that are controlled by exogenous (eg, feeding, sleep, stress, exercise) and endogenous (eg, gonadal, adrenal, thyroid hormones, hepatic and renal functions) originating stimuli.

Neurotransmitters responsible for the secretion of GHRH include direct stimuli through α_2-adrenergic neurons and indirect stimuli through changes in the secretion of SS. Dopamine and serotonin, by inhibiting SS, facilitate the effects that GHRH has in stimulating GH secretion. The stimulation of β_2-adrenergic neurons causes the secretion of SS and thus interferes with GH secretion (**Fig. 2**).

GH stimulation tests, whether physiologic or pharmacologic, help us understand the mechanisms whereby GH is secreted. Stimulation tests are used because basal GH is usually low. GH secretion can be stimulated physiologically (during sleep, after a meal,

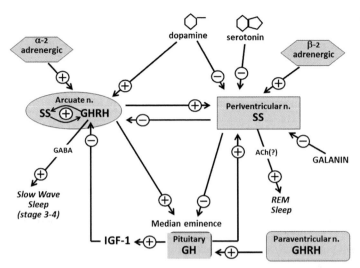

Fig. 2. The presumed roles of some of the principal neurotransmitters that control the secretion of GH through the interplay between GHRH and SS and their effects on some of the stages of sleep (*see text*).

or after strenuous exercise) or pharmacologically with a variety of agents that either stimulate specific centers in the CNS (α-adrenergic receptors in the ventromedial nucleus or arcuate nucleus of the hypothalamus) or alter metabolic homeostasis, creating stressful conditions (eg, hypoglycemia).

Because sleep disorders, feeding/weight, and linear growth have been associated in one manner or another with ADHD, all of which are directly or indirectly related to GH secretion, the following sections discuss if there may be any unifying concept to explain the association of these clinical manifestations with ADHD.

SLEEP, GH SECRETION, AND ADHD

That GH and sleep are associated can be appreciated from studies in such pathologic conditions as fatal familiar insomnia, in which the deterioration of sleep is associated with a decrease in GH secretion.[44] However, it has long been recognized that GH release increases during the night,[45] and nocturnal blood sampling for GH has been proposed as a diagnostic alternative to pharmacologic testing.

Studies that have determined frequent sampling (up to 30 seconds) and measurements of plasma GH levels combined with the deconvolution procedure, which mathematically estimates the rate of secretion of a hormone from the plasma concentrations, have revealed a close association of GH secretion with slow-wave sleep (SWS) as opposed to the lighter stages (stage 1 and 2) and rapid eye movement (REM) sleep.[46,47] Furthermore, secretion of GH and the amount of SWS both decrease in a similar fashion with advancing age.[48] However, although GH secretion occurs during SWS, it is believed that GH and SWS are not causally related but are generated by a common neural mechanism that may be related to the GH regulatory neuropeptide system.[49] This mechanism could be represented, at least in part, by GHRH, an endogenous 44 amino acid peptide with well-documented sleep-promoting activity[50] and which has also been shown to have a direct role in promoting non-REM sleep.[51–53]

In humans, intramuscular bolus injection of GH before the onset of sleep was found to increase REM sleep and to decrease SWS[54] probably by stimulating SS secretion, which has been shown to increase REM sleep in laboratory animals.[55] However, a subsequent study[56] failed to confirm this finding.

Several studies have looked into possible association between ADHD and sleep disturbances. The data suggest that some sleep disorders may be more common in ADHD. Like the problem with growth, there are similar controversies in trying to decide whether the sleep disorders observed in ADHD are an intrinsic part of the disorder, are related to another disorder that co-occurs with ADHD, or there is no relation, because more than 25% of all children have sleep disorders at some point.

A comparison between untreated children with ADHD and children without ADHD points to the following trends: (1) most studies show increased restlessness and periodic limb movement during sleep[57–60]; (2) other studies have suggested that sleep disturbances in ADHD could originate from the biochemical disturbances responsible for their deficits in attention and EF[61] and (3) still others have found that children with ADHD showed a lower cyclic alternating pattern (CAP) rate and a lower number of CAP sequences, supporting the hypothesis that sleep deprivation found in children with ADHD could be related to a dysregulation of arousal mechanisms and also play a role in the cause of ADHD.[58,62–64] However, a recent study[65] found no link between sleep patterns and ADHD, in that children with ADHD had no significant differences in CAP scoring compared with children without ADHD.

A study that looked at the polysomnographic sleep pattern of children with ADHD showed a significant increase in the duration of the absolute REM sleep and the number of sleep cycles when compared with controls. The overall pattern of the findings may reflect alterations of brain monoamines and cortical inhibitory control, presumably characteristic of ADHD.[66] A possible interpretation of these data might be that the low levels of dopamine described in ADHD could be responsible for decreased secretion of GHRH and removing its inhibitory effect on SS secretion. The combination of these 2 effects would lead to decreased SWS (low GHRH) and increased REM (increased SS) (see **Fig. 2**). Could this have repercussions on growth? The many controversial results produced in the literature, which may also reflect that ADHD may represent a variety of disorders, make this interpretation (or hypothesis) attractive but difficult to confirm.

WEIGHT, APPETITE/EATING, AND ADHD

In the next sections, both treated and nontreated children with ADHD are discussed in the hope that the information gathered can increase our understanding of the pathophysiology of ADHD. In addition, we cover some basic information regarding the neurotransmitter regulation of feeding to see if the weight changes described in the literature in both treated and nontreated patients could have a unifying explanation based on the currently accepted catecholamine hypothesis proposed to explain (at least in part) ADHD.

Weight of Untreated Patients with ADHD

Of the 3 characteristic components of ADHD, hyperactivity and impulsivity (which usually go together with or without inattentiveness) may be related to weight problems. Weight gain or loss is a function of energy intake (food) and energy expenditure (basal metabolism + degree of activity). It has been suggested that impulsivity may lead to the development of eating patterns that put children with ADHD at increased risk for obesity.[67,68] This possible explanation goes along with the research that linked overweight and ADD/ADHD.[69–71] According to most recent data obtained from the National Survey of Children's Health, which looked at anthropometric parameters of 46,707 individuals from 10 to 17 years of age, the prevalence of obesity and ADHD was 18.9% compared with 12.2% in apparently normal children/adolescents of the same age group.[72] In another study, untreated children and adolescents with ADHD had ~1.5 times the odds of being overweight, when compared with children and adolescents without ADHD.[73]

However, the hyperactive component of the disorder describes a child who cannot sit still and is constantly on the move (see **Box 1**), an individual who would not have adequate time to sit to eat ("fidgety Philip") and consumes more energy than a child of comparable age without ADHD. This characteristic of ADHD pushes the clinical picture towards one in which untreated children with ADHD are underweight, or at least not overweight/obese. This reasoning goes along with other data in the literature that have shown a decreased percent body fat and abdominal circumference (ie, clinical evidence of decreased nutritional status) in children with ADHD compared with population norms ($P<.01$).[74,75] Furthermore, because this finding was shown in both untreated and stimulant-treated children, it has been suggested that dysregulated growth may be caused by or at least associated with ADHD, independent of other factors.

However, aside from those studies that found untreated ADHD children to have decreased nutritional status, other studies found that untreated children with ADHD were of normal weight[76,77] and body mass index (BMI, calculated as weight in kilograms divided by the square of height in meters),[77,78] whereas still others found them to be heavier than normal.[79–83]

As can be appreciated from the controversial amount of information available, the reasoning process is not straightforward. Weight gain, or for that matter, weight maintenance or loss, depends on a multitude of variables, which include both genetic and environmental influences. This situation adds to the complexity of detecting a common clinical finding in children with ADHD, let alone finding a unifying cause to explain the contradictory reports on the weight status of untreated children with ADHD. Furthermore, because the pathophysiology of ADHD is poorly understood, it is probable that the ADHD population in many of the studies reported is heterogeneous. For this reason, a conclusive statement regarding the problem of weight is lacking.

Fig. 3 depicts a simplified hypothetical explanation of the pathophysiologic cause of the findings related to weight changes in untreated (and treated) children with ADHD.

Weight of Treated Patients with ADHD

The conventional, first-line medical treatment of children with ADHD has been with stimulant drugs. The most common drugs being used worldwide are methylphenidate and amphetamines. Although the mechanism of action of these drugs in ADHD is not known, the intrinsic characteristic of these drugs is to stimulate the release of catecholamines (dopamine and norepinephrine) from synapses of CNS neurons.

In analogy with the arguments presented in the section on weight of untreated patients with ADHD, it seems reasonable to hypothesize that the beneficial effect of medical treatment is to slow down the patient and make them focus more on what they are doing. Barring all the other variables involved in maintaining normal weight, the child who has been slowed down by medication and can now theoretically sit at the dinner table to eat may be expected to be in a favorable situation to gain weight. However, we must contend with some of the side effects of these drugs. Methylphenidate is a CNS stimulant, the action of which has been linked to inhibition of the DAT,

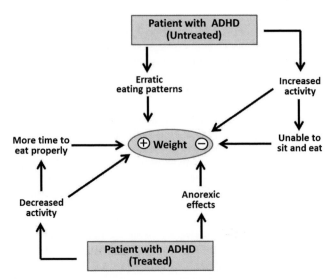

Fig. 3. Proposed influences that affect the nutritional-based behavior in untreated and treated ADHD. The figure emphasizes that in both the treated and the untreated patient with ADHD, there exist mechanisms that could theoretically account for either increased caloric intake or increased physical activity. It seems that the resulting clinical outcome depends on the interplay and predominant effect of these factors.

with consequent increases in dopamine made available for synaptic transmission. The important side effects of this drug, which may decrease the overall food intake, include its anorectic effect as well as effects on the gastrointestinal tract and abdominal pain. Dexamfetamine, a sympathomimetic amine, is also a central stimulant with adverse effects similar to methylphenidate. Atomoxetine, a selective noradrenaline reuptake inhibitor, also causes, among other things, decreased appetite, abdominal pain, nausea, and vomiting. Although these drugs have other and more important side effects, the list is limited to those that may deter a child being treated with these drugs from eating appropriately. Therefore, even though these drugs improve hyperactivity and impulsiveness and theoretically could ameliorate the nutritional situation, their important gastrointestinal/anorectic effects may prevail.

Approximately 70% to 80% of children with ADHD treated with stimulant medication experience significant relief from symptoms. In the remaining 20% to 30%, other drugs have been used such as tricyclic antidepressants (eg, imipramine), and α_2-adrenergic agonists (eg, clonidine and guanfacine). Again, the lack of a uniform response to these drugs indicates that we are potentially dealing with a heterogeneous group of conditions under the umbrella of ADHD.

Nevertheless, regarding the effect of stimulant medication on weight, there is more of a consensus, probably because weight loss is more a function of inadequate caloric intake (anorexic effects of the drugs) than of the beneficial effects on the hyperactivity. Most studies published concord that stimulant medications cause a significant decrease in weight.[78–81,83–91] The study of Waring and colleagues[73] found that treated children and adolescents with ADHD had ~1.6 times the odds of being underweight when compared with children and adolescents without ADHD.

Fig. 3 depicts a simplified hypothetical explanation of the pathophysiologic cause of the findings related to weight changes in treated (and untreated) children with ADHD.

Neurotransmitter Regulation of Appetite and Eating

Feeding is believed to be dependent on the balance between a feeding initiation system (eg, appetite) and a feeding cessation system (eg, satiety). The regulation of feeding is a complex process involving a variety of exogenous and endogenous inputs that are integrated within the CNS through neurotransmitter interactions that are interpreted as hunger or satiety. These neurotransmitter interactions take place primarily (but not exclusively) in specific areas of the CNS such as the paraventricular nucleus (PVN) or ventromedial hypothalamus (VMH) as well as in the region of the lateral hypothalamus (LH). The PVN seems to be the major defined system involving norepinephrine α-adrenergic transmission that is associated with the stimulation of feeding, whereas the LH, through β-adrenergic stimulation, is primarily involved with the inhibition of feeding. This system is held in check by satiety inputs coming from the PVN/VMH. This is an oversimplification of the intricate and complex interactions that occur both within the CNS and peripherally in the various organ systems as well as in the environment, which through a large number of neurotransmitters are capable of either initiating or inhibiting feeding. (**Fig. 4**)

In the next sections, some of the specific neurotransmitters involved in feeding are discussed, with reference to some (nonbiased) examples from the literature that could help us better understand the complexities occurring in the brain of a child with ADHD.

NOREPINEPHRINE

In a study of the neurochemical systems of the hypothalamus involved with feeding, one study found that α-adrenergic stimulation in the area of the PVN and VMH stimulated feeding, whereas β-adrenergic stimulation of the LH inhibited feeding.[92] However, whereas the effect of norepinephrine on the LH seems to be direct, as shown by studies indicating that injection of norepinephrine into the LH decreases feeding, and lesions in this area cause mild hyperphagia,[92] the effects on the PVN seem to be indirect. Lesions of the PVN have been shown to result in hyperphagia and to attenuate norepinephrine-induced eating.[93] This response suggests that the

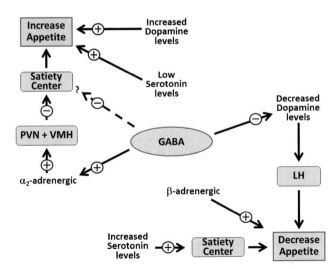

Fig. 4. Proposed involvement of neurotransmitters in the regulation of appetite and satiety (see text for explanation).

action of norepinephrine is secondary to the inhibition of the release of a satiety factor located in the PVN. One possible candidate for this satiety factor, which directly inhibits feeding, is corticotropin-releasing hormone, which in turn is inhibited by norepinephrine and stimulated by serotonin.[94]

SEROTONIN

Several studies have suggested that serotonin functions as a satiety center.[95] Depletion of brain serotonin by either neurotoxins (5,6-hydroxytryptamine) or serotonin synthesis depleters resulted in hyperphagia and obesity.[95] Serotonin agonists and drugs that potentiate serotonin actions (eg, fenfluramine) decrease feeding, whereas serotonin antagonists (eg, cyproheptadine) enhance feeding. Fenfluramine, a drug that increases serotonin content by stimulating synaptic release of serotonin and blocking its reuptake into presynaptic terminals, exerts a strong anorexigenic effect in both rodents and humans.[96] The effect of fenfluramine on food intake has been primarily attributed to serotonin action at 5-HT_{2C} receptors ($5\text{-HT}_{2C}R$) because the hypophagic responses induced by the drug are significantly blunted in $5\text{-HT}_{2C}R$ knockout mice.[97] Furthermore, because these $5\text{-HT}_{2C}R$ knockout mice also show hyperphagia and subsequently obesity, it has been suggested that the endogenous $5\text{-HT}_{2C}R$ are physiologic regulators of feeding and body weight.[98]

DOPAMINE

Several animal studies have shown that either destruction of dopaminergic and other catecholaminergic fibers with a specific neurotoxin (6-hydroxydopamine)[99–101] leads to hypophagia and weight loss. Dopamine-deficient (DD) mice, which cannot synthesize dopamine in dopaminergic neurons because of selective inactivation of the tyrosine hydroxylase gene, become hypoactive, hypophagic, and die of starvation by 4 weeks of age.[102] This inability to thrive was found to be caused by a failure of normal dopamine signaling rather than aberrant neural development.[102] Studies that restored dopamine production in the caudate putamen of these mice also restored feeding.[103]

Additional information that implicates the importance of the dopaminergic system in feeding was obtained by Szczypka and colleagues,[104] who showed that injections of L-dopa in DD mice elicit an intense period of feeding that lasts a few hours, gradually subsiding as the dopamine produced from the L-dopa is metabolized. As the dopamine content decreased to approximately 4% of normal (occurring in approximately 6–9 hours), DD mice failed to eat enough to sustain themselves and died within 48 hours.[104]

GABA

GABA is the major inhibitory neurotransmitter in the brain, occurring in 30% to 40% of all synapses, and is intricately connected to both the norepinephrine and dopaminergic neurotransmitter systems. Norepinephrine-induced feeding (α-adrenergic stimulation) (see earlier discussion) is inhibited by GABA antagonists. This finding suggests that the α-adrenergic feeding system may operate through stimulation of GABA release, which in turn inhibits the release of the satiety factor from the PVN.[105,106] When GABA is injected into the nigrostriated tracts, it inhibits feeding, possibly by reducing dopaminergic transmission from the substantia nigra. It seems that this universal inhibitory neurotransmitter increases appetite by inhibiting the satiety center and its neurologic connections and decreases food intake by inhibiting the lateral hypothalamic dopaminergic system.

If all of the animal studies cited earlier were transferred to the child with ADHD, who supposedly lacks adequate amounts of the indicated neurotransmitter in key areas of the brain, they would imply that these children should express a certain degree of anorexia and this together with the hyperactivity should create a milieu conducive of weight loss or, at the most, weight maintenance but not obesity (see **Figs. 3** and **4**). However, the argument is complex, and this information can only put ADHD under a different, more complex, light.

GROWTH, PUBERTY, AND ADHD

Although concerns regarding growth deficits in children with ADHD date back more than 40 years,[107] despite the numerous articles that have appeared in the literature, there continues to be no consensus on whether ADHD is associated with poor growth or whether adrenergic stimulant treatment affects linear growth. A first step in approaching this question is to review the current information that exists concerning the normal pattern of growth of untreated children with ADHD, and, in addition, to understand if and how the neurotransmitter abnormalities described in ADHD could affect growth in the native state or under the effects of stimulant treatment.

According to **Fig. 2**, which summarizes the current information regarding GH secretion, the presence of dopamine is important in stimulating GH secretion because of its direct stimulatory action on the secretion of GHRH and indirect action on its inhibitory effect on SS secretion. Likewise, α_2-adrenergic stimulation, through norepinephrine, is also important in its stimulatory effect on GHRH secretion. Serotonin could also influence GH secretion, indirectly, by its inhibiting effect on SS secretion. It therefore seems that all 3 of the neurotransmitters that have been described to be deficient in the CNS of children with ADHD are directly or indirectly related to GH secretion and supposedly the growth that ensues. Therefore, in the untreated state, the child with ADHD could lack the appropriate stimulants to favor the internal environmental conditions that are conducive to normal growth.

GROWTH AND PUBERTY OF UNTREATED PATIENTS

A review of the literature concerning the growth of untreated children with ADHD shows that no single pattern seems to be encountered in this disorder. Although the usual contention has been that untreated children with ADHD usually have height deficits, which have been proposed to be caused by, or at least associated with, the disease,[74,75,108] other studies found that untreated children were of normal height,[77,79] whereas still others found these children to be taller than normal.[80–82,88,89]

An important aspect in the evaluation of linear growth is the determination of bone age. A review of the literature looking for correlations between bone age and growth in children with ADHD was disappointing. We were able to find only 2 articles, both more than 30 years old. In 1974, Oettinger and colleagues[109] looked at the bone ages of 53 children (43 boys) with what then was referred to as MBD. The purpose of this study was to confirm whether or not the opinion of parents and teachers that these children were more immature than their peers had a biological reason. These investigators found that bone ages in children with MBD was significantly retarded ($P<.01$) compared with the standards group's norms. Two-thirds were less than the mean and almost 20% showed a bone age of more than 2 standard deviations (SD) less than the mean. In 1979, Schlager and colleagues[110] studied the skeletal maturation of 60 children (45 boys) with MBD and found the mean bone age to be more than 8 months lower than the mean chronologic age, with 10% of the group having an SD more than 2 less than the mean for age. The bone age information lends support to the usually accepted idea that untreated children with ADHD are shorter than their peers, and could indirectly imply that the delayed bone age is responsible for the height deficit.

Information in the literature that could help confirm this association is also contradictory. Articles that would be in line with the delayed bone age finding have reported that height deficits in untreated children with ADHD are found only in early adolescent-aged boys and that this early adolescent growth delay spontaneously improves by late adolescence or early adulthood with no apparent effect on adult stature.[109,110] However, if these conclusions were correct, some evidence would be expected that these children manifest delayed onset of puberty. According to a recent report that compared the age of pubertal onset of untreated and treated boys with ADHD, no such evidence was found.[111] Boys taking stimulant medication had a mean age of 10.1 years (confidence interval [CI], 9.6–10.6) when testicular volume reached a size greater than 3 mL, whereas untreated children had a mean age of 9.8 years (CI, 9.7–10.0). Although these results suggest that there is no difference in the age of pubertal onset between untreated and treated children with ADHD, no information is given regarding whether these children did or did not have evidence of growth delay.

The conclusion that seems to stand out from all of the articles reviewed is that a methodologic comparison of the various published studies is, most of the time, difficult to perform. This difficulty is because of a lack of well-organized prospective, longitudinal, holistic investigations that methodically study the problem of growth from all aspects, both from an intrinsic (growth velocities, bone maturation, pubertal development) and extrinsic (the genetic and environmental factors, which are important variables in the process of reaching adult stature) perspective.

GROWTH AND PUBERTY OF TREATED PATIENTS

Most of the existing literature on growth and ADHD deals with the effects of the commonly used medical treatment in this disorder. However, there is a lot of controversy as to whether these drugs cause poor growth[76,81,84–91,107,112–114] or not[77,79,115,116] and what the underlying mechanisms may be in cases in which growth is affected. Nevertheless, reductions in height are commonly reported with stimulant therapy use for ADHD, with an estimated height deficit between 1 and 3 cm, averaging approximately 1 cm/y over a 3-year period.[84,107,117,118] Although treated patients may suffer from the anorexic effects of the drugs used and may be associated with some degree of weight loss, no association has been reported between weight loss and height deficits. Furthermore, observed growth deficits do not seem to be associated with pubertal delay[111] nor do they seem to interfere with the attainment of normal adult height even if therapy may have had an adverse effect on children's growth rate.[119,120]

Several studies have reported that children who had height suppression caused by prolonged stimulant treatment manifested a rebound growth acceleration after interruption of the drug.[84,85,118,120,121] However, other studies have shown catch-up growth in height during treatment.[85,115,122] These discrepant results are difficult to interpret and consequently some have suggested that the stimulant-associated height deficits reported in ADHD might be temporary and early manifestations of the disorder and not complications of treatment.[117]

This apparent cause and effect relationship between suspension of therapy and catch-up growth could also imply that treatment somehow interferes with the normal process of growth and that with the discontinuation of this treatment, the body tries to return to the previous growth pattern by showing catch-up growth. This finding contradicts the presumed, neurotransmitter-responsible growth schema indicated in **Fig. 2**, which instead explains the catch-up growth during treatment. A possible unifying explanation could be that because ADHD is not a single entity, but possibly a continuum of qualitative and quantitative neurotransmitter defects/deficiency, the increase in neurotransmitter levels resulting from the treatment, in an individual not accustomed to such levels may cause a downregulation of those receptors that are involved with the neurotransmitter regulation of GH secretion. This hypothesis is strictly conjectural because no such studies have been found in the literature. The catch-up growth observed at the suspension of treatment could be a manifestation of a return to a normal pretreatment state, whereas the catch-up growth observed during treatment may be occurring in individuals whose neurotransmitter levels have increased sufficiently but not excessively.

RESPONSE TO GROWTH HARMONE IN CHILDREN WITH ADHD

From an analysis of Genentech's National Cooperative Growth Study (NCGS) database of children receiving GH, Frindik and colleagues[123] report that close to 6% of the more than 12000 children enrolled were receiving ADHD medications. However, no information is available as to how many patients with ADHD not receiving specific medication are being treated with GH. Therefore, because of the potentially, rather high percentage of children with ADHD receiving GH, this article would not be complete without addressing the question of how children with ADHD respond to growth hormone treatment, whether or not they are being treated with stimulant medications.

Unfortunately we were not able to find any articles of GH replacement in children with ADHD not on stimulant medication. However, in line with what has been previously discussed in this article, it could be inferred that GH treatment would directly by-pass any potentially altered mechanism existing in children with ADHD that could be responsible for appropriate GH secretion and therefore one should see no differences between GH-treated short stature patients and ADHD patients.

With regard to patients with ADHD on stimulant medication, the few papers that have been published looking at the GH response in these children challenges the belief that such children do not seem to respond as well to GH as children receiving only GH. Frindlik and colleagues[123] found that first year growth rates in idiopathic short stature (ISS) ADHD patients (8.1 ± 1.9 cm; mean ± sd) were similar to those of ISS subjects (8.6 ± 2.1 cm) and concluded that ADHD treatment did not interfere with the growth response to GH. Rao and colleagues[124] using a stepwise multiple regression method, looked at stimulant-treated ADHD patients and compared the GH response of ADHD patients who had isolated growth hormone deficiency (IGHD) (n = 184) with IGHD subjects (n = 2313) and ADHD patients with idiopathic short stature (ISS) (n = 117) with ISS subjects(n = 1283). These authors found that the use of stimulant medication had a small negative effect on the change in height SDS in the ADHD-IGHD which decreased with time when compared to the IGHD patients; whereas, in the ISS cohort, stimulant medication had no demonstrative effect on the response to GH therapy.

From these limited studies, it would appear that the growth response of children with ADHD who need to be treated with GH does not differ from other children requiring the hormone.

SUMMARY

The discrepancies that have been documented in the literature over the last 40 years regarding growth in ADHD and in its treatment make this argument one that is still riddled by confusion and controversy. The enormous variabilities that have been described, whether in treated or untreated children with ADHD, imply that we are not dealing with a single entity but probably varying degrees or expressions of the disorder or its treatment (response to different medications and the use of different doses of the same medication). This renders any attempt to answer the original question regarding growth and ADHD as a taxing endeavor that would be open to criticism based on the amount of nonconclusive information that has been printed over the last 50 years or more.

However, the review of this argument does allow for some conclusions and suggestions to be made. One of the major conclusions is that most of the studies are not comparable for several reasons: (1) different methods of assessing growth, (2) consistent lack of adequate information to assess final growth potential, (3) lack of sound scientific evidence regarding associations between growth, bone age, maturation, and pubertal development, (4) comparison between different age groups, (5) the use of different medications, and (6) different doses of the same medication. If all of these variables are further considered within the context of the possible variability in the expression of the disorder, we may spend the next 50 years continuing these controversies, all perfectly legitimate, and still not clarify the problem. These conclusions suggest that we need to conduct well-organized studies that are prospective, longitudinal, and approached from a multidisciplinary aspect in order to cover the most important variables that could give us a definitive answer.

Nevertheless, a tentative attempt to unify all of the controversial data that are found in the literature with the premise that each published article has been conducted in a methodologically correct manner and that the results presented indicate ADHD could imply that each of the results presented, even if appearing contradictory, may be one of the many expressions of the disorder that could be explained by the qualitative and quantitative degree of CNS involvement of neurotransmitter deficiencies.

One last and important consideration is that the improvement obtained from the medications in a child's social, educational, and overall quality of life outweighs and overshadows any temporary growth problem that may be encountered during therapy.

REFERENCES

1. Brown TE. ADD/ADHD and impaired executive function in clinical practice. Current Attention Disorders Reports 2009;1:37–41. http://dx.doi.org/10.1007/s12618-009-0006-3.

2. Crichton A. An inquiry into the nature and origin of mental derangement. On attention and its diseases. J Atten Disord 2008;12:200–4.

3. Heinrich H. "Struwwelpeter" (English translation). New York: Dover Publications; 1995. ISBN 9780486284699.

4. Still GF. The Goulstonian lectures on "Some abnormal psychical conditions in children". Lancet 1902;1:1008–12.

5. Bradley C. The behavior of children receiving benzedrine. Am J Psychiatry 1937;94:577–88.

6. Clements SD, Peters JE. Minimal brain dysfunctions in the school-age child. Diagnosis and treatment. Arch Gen Psychiatry 1962;6:185–97.

7. International statistical classification of diseases and related health problems, 10th revision. 2nd edition. Geneva: World Health Organization; 2010.

8. Polanczyk G, Silva de Lima M, Lessa Horta B, et al. The worldwide prevalence of ADHD: a systematic review and metaregression analysis. Am J Psychiatry 2007;164:942–8.

9. Anderson JC. Is childhood hyperactivity the product of Western culture? Lancet 1996;348:73–4.

10. Timini S, Taylor E. ADHD is best understood as a cultural construct. Br J Psychiatry 2004;184:8–9.

11. American Psychiatric Association. Diagnostic and statistical manual of mental disorders (DSM-4). 4th edition. Washington, DC: American Psychiatric Press; 2000.

12. Agency for Healthcare Research and Quality. Diagnosis of attention-deficit/hyperactivity disorder. Clinical Focus. Rockville (MD): Agency for Healthcare Research and Quality; 1999. Available at: http://archive.ahrq.gov/clinic/tp/adhddtp.htm.

13. Willcutt EG, Pennington BF. Comorbidity of reading disability and attention-deficit/hyperactivity disorder: differences by gender and subtype. J Learn Disabil 2000;33:179–91.

14. Sax L, Kautz KJ. Who suggests the diagnosis of attention-deficit/hyperactivity disorder? Ann Fam Med 2003;1:171–4.

15. National Institute for Health and Clinical Excellence. Attention deficit hyperactivity disorder–diagnosis and management of ADHD in children, young people and adults. Nice Clinical Guideline 72, September 2008. Available at: http://www.nice.org.uk/nicemedia/live/12061/42059/42059.pdf.

16. Angold A, Erkanli A, Egger HL, et al. Stimulant treatment for children: a community perspective. J Am Acad Child Adolesc Psychiatry 2000;39:975–84.

17. Scheffler RM, Hinshaw SP, Modrek S, et al. The global market for ADHD medications. Health Aff 2007;26(2):450–7.

18. Chai G, Governale L, McMahon AW, et al. Trends of outpatient prescription drug utilization in US children, 2002-2010. Pediatrics 2012;130:23–31.

19. Biederman J, Faraone S. Attention-deficit hyperactivity disorder. Lancet 2005; 366:237–48.

20. Goodman R, Stevenson J. A twin study of hyperactivity. II. The aetiological role of genes, family relationships and perinatal adversity. J Child Psychol Psychiatry 1989;30:691–709.

21. Sprich S, Biederman J, Crawford M, et al. Adoptive and biological families of children and adolescents with ADHD. J Am Acad Child Adolesc Psychiatry 2000;39:1432–7.

22. Faraone SV, Biederman J, Friedman D. Validity of DSM-IV subtypes of attention-deficit/ hyperactivity disorder: a family study perspective. J Am Acad Child Adolesc Psychiatry 2000;39:300–7.

23. Biederman J, Faraone SV, Keenan K, et al. Family-genetic and psychosocial risk factors in DSM-III attention deficit disorder. J Am Acad Child Adolesc Psychiatry 1990;29:526–33.

24. Walcott CM, Landau S. The relation between disinhibition and emotion regulation in boys with attention deficit hyperactivity disorder. J Clin Child Adolesc Psychol 2004;33(4):772–82.

25. Lou HC, Henriksen L, Bruhn P. Focal cerebral hypoperfusion in children with dysphasia and/or attention deficit disorder. Arch Neurol 1984;41:825–9.

26. Lou HC, Henriksen L, Bruhn P, et al. Striatal dysfunction in attention deficit and hyperkinetic disorder. Arch Neurol 1989;46:48–52.

27. Lou HC, Henriksen L, Bruhn P. Focal cerebral dysfunction in developmental learning disabilities. Lancet 1990;335:8–11.

28. Zametkin AJ, Nordahl TE, Gross M, et al. Cerebral glucose metabolism in adults with hyperactivity of childhood onset. N Engl J Med 1990;323:1361–6.

29. Valera EM, Faraone SV, Murray KE, et al. Meta-analysis of structural imaging findings in attention-deficit/hyperactivity disorder. Biol Psychiatry 2007;61:1361–9.

30. Durston S, Tottenham NT, Thomas KM, et al. Differential patterns of striatal activation in young children with and without ADHD. Biol Psychiatry 2003;53: 871–8.

31. Ellison-Wright I, Ellison-Wright Z, Bullmore E. Structural brain change in attention deficit hyperactivity disorder identified by meta-analysis. BMC Psychiatry 2008; 8:51–8.

32. Barry RJ, Clarke AR, Johnstone SJ. A review of electrophysiology in attention-deficit/hyperactivity disorder: I. Qualitative and quantitative electro-encephalography. Clin Neurophysiol 2003;114:171–83.

33. Asherson P. Attention-deficit hyperactivity disorder in the post-genomic era. Eur Child Adolesc Psychiatry 2004;13(Suppl 1):I50–70.

34. Faraone SV, Perlis RH, Doyle AE, et al. Molecular genetics of attention-deficit/hyperactivity disorder. Biol Psychiatry 2005;57(11):1313–23.

35. Magara F, Ricceri L, Wolfer DP, et al. The acallosal mouse strain I/LnJ: a putative model of ADHD? Neurosci Biobehav Rev 2000;24:45–50.

36. Shaywitz SE, Cohen DJ, Shaywitz BA. The biochemical basis of minimal brain dysfunction. J Pediatr 1978;92:179–87.

37. Russell V, de Villiers A, Sagvolden T, et al. Altered dopaminergic function in the prefrontal cortex, nucleus accumbens and caudate-putamen of an animal model of attention-deficit hyperactivity disorder: the spontaneously hypertensive rat. Brain Res 1995;676:343–51.

38. Rubinstein M, Phillips TJ, Bunzow JR, et al. Mice lacking dopamine D4 receptors are supersensitive to ethanol, cocaine, and methamphetamine. Cell 1997; 90:991–1001.

39. Dulawa SC, Grandy DK, Low MJ, et al. Dopamine D4 receptor- knock-out mice exhibit reduced exploration of novel stimuli. J Neurosci 1999;19:9550–6.

40. Gainetdinov RR, Wetsel WC, Jones SR, et al. Role of serotonin in the paradoxical calming effect of psychostimulants on hyperactivity. Science 1999;283:397–402.

41. Giros B, Jaber M, Jones SR, et al. Hyperlocomotion and indifference to cocaine and amphetamine in mice lacking the dopamine transporter. Nature 1996;379: 606–12.

42. Zametkin AJ, Rapoport JL. Neurobiology of attention deficit disorder with hyperactivity: where have we come in 50 years? J Am Acad Child Adolesc Psychiatry 1987;26:676–86.

43. Dougherty DD, Bonab AA, Spencer TJ, et al. Dopamine transporter density is elevated in patients with attention deficit hyperactivity disorder. Lancet 1999; 354:2132–3.

44. Portaluppi F, Cortelli P, Avoni P, et al. Dissociated 24-hour patterns of somatotropin and prolactin in fatal familiar insomnia. Neuroendocrinology 1995;61:731–7.

45. Takahashi Y, Kipnis M, Daughday WH. Growth hormone secretion during sleep. J Clin Invest 1968;47:2079–90.

46. Holl RW, Hartman ML, Veldhuis JD, et al. Thirty-second sampling of plasma growth hormone in man: correlation with sleep stages. J Clin Endocrinol Metab 1991;72:854–61.

47. Van Cauter E, Kerkhofs M, Caufriez A, et al. A quantitative estimation of growth hormone secretion in normal man: reproducibility and relation to sleep and time of day. J Clin Endocrinol Metab 1992;74:1441–50.

48. Van Cauter E, Plat L, Copinschi G. Interrelations between sleep and somatotropic axis. Sleep 1998;21:553–66.

49. Steiger A, Guldner J, Hemmeter U, et al. Effects of growth-hormone releasing hormone on sleep EEG and nocturnal hormone secretion in male controls. Neuroendocrinology 1992;56:566–73.
50. Steiger A. Sleep and endocrinology. J Intern Med 2003;254:13–22.
51. Steiger A, Guldner J, Hemmeter U, et al. Effects of growth hormone-releasing hormone and somatostatin on sleep EEG and nocturnal hormone secretion in male controls. Neuroendocrinology 1992;56:566–73.
52. Marshall L, Mölle M, Böschen G, et al. Greater efficacy of episodic than continuous growth hormone releasing hormone (GHRH) administration in promoting slow-wave sleep (SWS). J Clin Endocrinol Metab 1996;81:1009–13.
53. Obal F, Krueger JM. GHRH and sleep. Sleep Med Rev 2004;8(5):367–77.
54. Mendelson WB, Slater S, Gold P, et al. The effect of growth hormone administration on human sleep: a dose-response study. Biol Psychiatry 1980;15:613–8.
55. Danguir J. Intracerebroventricular infusion of somatostatin selectively increases paradoxical sleep in rats. Brain Res 1986;367:26–30.
56. Kern W, Halder R, Al-Reda S, et al. Systemic growth hormone does not affect human sleep. J Clin Endocrinol Metab 1993;76:1428–32.
57. Cortese S, Konofal E, Lecendreux M, et al. Restless leg syndrome and attention-deficit/hyperactivity disorder: a review of the literature. Sleep 2005;28:1007–13.
58. Golan N, Shahar E, Ravid S, et al. Sleep disorders and daytime sleepiness in children with attention-deficit/hyperactivity disorder. Sleep 2004;27:261–6.
59. Corkum P, Tannock R, Moldofksy H. Sleep disturbances in children with attention-deficit/hyperactivity disorder. J Am Acad Child Adolesc Psychiatry 1998;37:637–46.
60. O'Brien LM, Gozal D. Sleep in children with attention-deficit/hyperactivity disorder. Minerva Pediatr 2004;56:585–601.
61. Cohen-Zion M, Ancoli-Israel S. Sleep in children with attention-deficit hyperactivity disorder (ADHD): a review of naturalistic and stimulant intervention studies. Sleep Med Rev 2004;8:379–402.
62. Ramos Platon MJ, Vela Bueno A, Espinar Sierra J, et al. Hypnopolygraphic alterations in attention deficit disorder (ADD) children. Int J Neurosci 1990;53:87–101.
63. Lecendreux M, Konofal E, Bouvard M, et al. Sleep and alertness in children with ADHD. J Child Psychol Psychiatry 2000;41:803–12.
64. Miano S, Donfrancesco R, Bruni O, et al. NREM sleep instability is reduced in children with attention-deficit/hyperactivity disorder. Sleep 2006;29(6):797–803.
65. Príhodová I, Paclt I, Kemlink D, et al. Sleep microstructure is not altered in children with attention-deficit/hyperactivity disorder (ADHD). Psychol Res 2012;61(1):125–33.
66. Kirov R, Kinkelbur J, Heipke S, et al. Is there a specific polysomnographic sleep pattern in children with attention deficit/hyperactivity disorder. J Sleep Res 2004;13:87–93.
67. Barkley RA, McMurray MB, Edelbrock CS, et al. Side effects of methylphenidate in children with attention deficit hyperactivity disorder: a system, placebo-controlled evaluation. Pediatrics 1990;86(2):184–92.
68. Agranat-Meged AN, Deitcher C, Goldzweig G, et al. Childhood obesity and attention deficit/hyperactivity disorder: a newly described comorbidity in obese hospitalized children. Int J Eat Disord 2005;37(4):357–9.
69. Holtkamp K, Konrad K, Muller B, et al. Overweight and obesity in children with attention-deficit/hyperactivity disorder. Int J Obes Relat Metab Disord 2004;28(5):685–9.

70. Hubel R, Jass J, Marcus A, et al. Overweight and basal metabolic rate in boys with attention-deficit/hyperactivity disorder. Eat Weight Disord 2006;11(3): 139–46.

71. Bandini LG, Curtin C, Hamad C, et al. Prevalence of overweight in children with developmental disorders in the continuous National Health and Nutrition Examination Survey (NHANES) 1999–2002. J Pediatr 2005;146(6):738–43.

72. Chen AY, Kim SE, Houtrow AJ, et al. Prevalence of obesity among children with chronic conditions. Obesity (Silver Spring) 2010;18(1):210–3.

73. Waring ME, Kate MA, Lapane L. Overweight in children and adolescents in relation to attention-deficit/hyperactivity disorder: results from a national sample. Pediatrics 2008;122:e1–6.

74. Ptacek R, Kuzelova H, Pactl I, et al. Anthropometric changes in non-medicated ADHD boys. Neuro Endocrinol Lett 2009;30(3):377–81.

75. Ptacek R, Kuzelova H, Pactl I, et al. ADHD and growth: anthropometric changes in medicated and non-medicated ADHD boys. Med Sci Monit 2009;15(12):595–9.

76. Roche AF, Lipman RS, Overall JE, et al. The effects of stimulant medication on the growth of hyperkinetic children. Pediatrics 1979;63(6):847–50.

77. Bereket A, Turan S, Karaman MG, et al. Height, weight, IGF-1, IGFBP-3 and thyroid functions in prepubertal children with attention deficit hyperactivity disorder: effect of methylphenidate treatment. Horm Res 2005;63:159–64.

78. Zachor DA, Roberts AW, Hodgens JB, et al. Effects of long-term psychostimulant medication on growth of children with ADHD. Res Dev Disabil 2006;27: 162–74.

79. Spencer TJ, Faraone SV, Biederman J, et al. Does prolonged therapy with a long-acting stimulant suppress growth in children with ADHD? J Am Acad Child Adolesc Psychiatry 2006;45(5):527–37.

80. Faraone SV, Biederman J, Morley CP, et al. Effect of stimulants on height and weight: a review of the literature. J Am Acad Child Adolesc Psychiatry 2008; 47(9):994–1009.

81. Poulton A, Cowell CT. Slowing of growth in height and weight on stimulants: a characteristic pattern. J Paediatr Child Health 2003;39:180–5.

82. MTA Cooperative Group. National Institute of Mental Health multimodal treatment study of ADHD follow-up: changes in effectiveness and growth after the end of treatment. Pediatrics 2004;113(4):762–9.

83. Sund AM, Zeiner P. Does extended medication with amphetamine or methylphenidate reduce growth in hyperactive children? Nord J Psychiatry 2002;56(1): 53–7.

84. Safer DJ, Allen RP. Factors influencing the suppressant effects of two stimulant drugs on the growth of hyperactive children. Pediatrics 1973;51(4):660–7.

85. Satterfield JH, Cantwell DP, Schell A, et al. Growth of hyperactive children treated with methylphenidate. Arch Gen Psychiatry 1979;36(2):212–7.

86. Loney J, Whaley-Klahn MA, Ponto LB, et al. Predictors of adolescent height and weight in hyperkinetic boys treated with methylphenidate [proceedings]. Psychopharmacol Bull 1981;17(1):132–4.

87. Poulton A. Growth on stimulant medication; clarifying the confusion: a review. Arch Dis Child 2005;90:801–6.

88. Swanson J, Greenhill L, Wigal T, et al. Stimulant-related reductions of growth rates in the PATS. J Am Acad Child Adolesc Psychiatry 2006;45(11):1304–13.

89. Swanson JM, Elliott GR, Greenhill LL, et al. Effects of stimulant medication on growth rates across 3 years in the MTA follow-up. J Am Acad Child Adolesc Psychiatry 2007;46(8):1015–27.

90. Faraone SV, Giefer EE. Long-term effects of methylphenidate transdermal delivery system treatment of ADHD on growth. J Am Acad Child Adolesc Psychiatry 2007;46(9):1138–47.
91. Faraone SV, Spencer TJ, Kollins SH, et al. Effects of lisdexamfetamine dimesylate treatment for ADHD on growth. J Am Acad Child Adolesc Psychiatry 2010; 49(1):24–32.
92. Leibovitz SF. Neurochemical systems of the hypothalamus in control of feeding and drinking behaviour and water and electrolyte excretion. In: Morgone P, Panksepp J, editors. Handbook of the hypothalamus, vol. 3. New York: Marcel-Dekker; 1980. p. 299–437.
93. Leibovitz SF, Hammer NJ, Chang K. Feeding behaviour induced by central norepinephrine injection is attenuated by discrete lesions in the hypothalamic paraventricular nucleus. Pharmacol Biochem Behav 1983;19:945–50.
94. Buckingham JC. Corticotropin releasing factor. Pharmacol Rev 1980;31:253–74.
95. Blundell JE. Serotonin and feeding. In: Esmon WR, editor. Serotonin in health and disease, vol. 5. New York: Spectrum; 1979. p. 403–50.
96. McGuirk J, Goodall E, Silverstone T, et al. Differential effects of d-fenfluramine, l-fenfluramine and d-amphetamine on the microstructure of human eating behaviour. Behav Pharmacol 1991;2:113–9.
97. Vickers SP, Clifton PG, Dourish CT, et al. Reduced satiating effect of fenfluramine in serotonin 5-HT(2C) receptor mutant mice. Psychopharmacology (Berl) 1999; 143:309–14.
98. Nonogaki K, Strack AM, Dallman MF, et al. Leptin-independent hyperphagia and type 2 diabetes in mice with a mutated serotonin 5-HT2C receptor gene. Nat Med 1998;4:1152–6.
99. Zigmond MJ, Stricker EM. Deficits in feeding behavior after intraventricular injection of 6-hydroxydopamine in rats. Science 1972;177:1211–4.
100. Nadaud D, Simon H, Herman JP, et al. Contributions of the mesencephalic dopaminergic system and the trigeminal sensory pathway to the ventral tegmental aphagia syndrome in rats. Physiol Behav 1984;33(6):879–87.
101. Lénárd L, Jandó G, Karádi Z, et al. Lateral hypothalamic feeding mechanisms: iontophoretic effects of kainic acid, ibotenic acid and 6-hydroxydopamine. Brain Res Bull 1988;20(6):847–56.
102. Zhou QY, Palmiter RD. Dopamine-deficient mice are severely hypoactive, adipsic and aphagic. Cell 1995;83:1197–209.
103. Szczypka MS, Kwok K, Brot MD, et al. Dopamine production in the caudate putamen restores feeding in dopamine-deficient mice. Neuron 2001;30: 819–28.
104. Szczypka MS, Rainey MA, Kim DS, et al. Feeding behavior in dopamine-deficient mice. Proc Natl Acad Sci U S A 1999;96:12138–43.
105. Panksepp J, Bishop P, Rossi J III. Neurohumoral and endocrine control of feeding. Psychoneuroendocrinology 1979;4:89–106.
106. Morley JF, Levine AS, Kneip J. Muscimol induced feeding. A model to study the hypothalamic regulation of appetite. Life Sci 1981;29:1213–8.
107. Safer D, Allen R, Barr E. Depression of growth in hyperactive children on stimulant drugs. N Engl J Med 1972;287:217–20.
108. Spencer T, Biederman J, Harding M, et al. Growth deficits on ADHD children revisited: evidence for disorder-associated growth delays? J Am Acad Child Adolesc Psychiatry 1996;35(11):1460–9.
109. Oettinger L Jr, Majovski LV, Limbeck GA, et al. Bone age in children with minimal brain dysfunction. Percept Mot Skills 1974;39:1127–31.

110. Schlager G, Newman DE, Dunn HG, et al. Bone age in children with minimal brain dysfunction. Dev Med Child Neurol 1979;21:41–51.
111. Steffes JM, Slora EJ, Hussey M, et al. Age of pubertal onset of boys taking stimulant medications. Presented at the Pediatric Academic Societies. Denver Colorado, April 30–May 3, 2011.
112. Mattes JA, Gittelman R. Growth of hyperactive children on maintenance regimen of methylphenidate. Arch Gen Psychiatry 1983;40(3):317–21.
113. Greenhill LL, Puig-Antich J, Novacenko H, et al. Prolactin, growth hormone and growth responses in boys with attention hyperactivity disorder and hyperactivity treated with methylphenidate. J Am Acad Child Psychiatry 1984;23(1):58–67.
114. Lisska MC, Rivkees SA. Daily methylphenidate use slows the growth of children, a community based study. J Pediatr Endocrinol Metab 2003;16(5):711–8.
115. Gross MD. Growth of hyperkinetic children taking methylphenidate, dextroamphetamine, or imipramine/desipramine. Pediatrics 1976;58(3):423–31.
116. Millichap JG. Growth of hyperactive children treated with methylphenidate. J Learn Disabil 1978;11(9):567–70.
117. Spencer T, Biederman J, Wilens T. Growth deficits in children with attention deficit hyperactivity disorder. Pediatrics 1998;102:501–6.
118. Safer D, Allen R, Barr E. Growth rebound after termination of stimulant drugs. J Pediatr 1975;86:113–6.
119. Hechtman L, Weiss G, Perlman T. Young adult outcome of hyperactive children who received long-term stimulant treatment. J Am Acad Child Psychiatry 1984; 23:261–9.
120. Gittelman R, Mannuzza S. Hyperactive boys almost grown up. III. Methylphenidate effects on ultimate height. Arch Gen Psychiatry 1988;45:1131–4.
121. Gittelman R, Landa B, Mattes J, et al. Methylphenidate and growth in hyperactive children. Arch Gen Psychiatry 1988;45:1127–30.
122. Dickinson LC, Lee J, Ringdahl IC, et al. Impaired growth in hyperkinetic children receiving pemoline. Pediatrics 1979;94:538–41.
123. Frindik JP, Morales A, Fowlkes J, et al. Stimulant medication use and response to growth hormone therapy : An NCGS database analysis. Horm Res 2009;72: 160–6.
124. Rao JK, Julius JR, Breen TJ, et al. Response to growth hormone in attention deficit hyperactivity disorder: Effects of methyphenidate and pemoline therapy. Pediatrics 1998;102:497–500.

Safety of Growth Hormone Treatment in Patients Previously Treated for Cancer

Wassim Chemaitilly, MD[a],*, Leslie L. Robison, PhD[b]

KEYWORDS

- Growth hormone deficiency • Childhood cancer survivor • Cancer recurrence
- Second neoplasms • Cancer survivors

KEY POINTS

- The use of growth hormone (GH) in cancer survivors raises safety concerns because of the mitogenic and proliferative properties of GH and insulin-like growth factor 1 (IGF-1).
- Treatment with GH in childhood cancer survivors has not been shown to increase the risks of disease recurrence or mortality.
- Treatment with GH may be associated with an increased risk of second neoplasms, but studies are based on a few events.
- Radiation-associated meningiomas are the most common second neoplasms observed in GH-treated individuals.
- Exposure to cranial radiotherapy also predisposes to the development of meningiomas.
- Cancer survivors treated with GH require close monitoring during therapy and long-term follow-up.
- More data are needed on the long-term safety and benefits of GH replacement in deficient adult survivors.

INTRODUCTION

GH deficiency (GHD) is one of the most commonly observed hormonal disorders in brain tumors survivors. Patients with tumor development close to the hypothalamus and/or pituitary and, more commonly, individuals exposed to cranial radiotherapy are particularly at risk of GHD.[1] Contemporary regimens of GH replacement therapy are effective in restoring linear growth and improving the adult height outcomes of

Conflict of interest: Dr Chemaitilly—None; Dr Robison—Consultant for Eli Lilly.
[a] Division of Endocrinology, Department of Pediatric Medicine, St Jude Children's Research Hospital, 262 Danny Thomas Place, MS 737, Memphis, TN 38105-3678, USA; [b] Department of Epidemiology and Cancer Control, St Jude Children's Research Hospital, 262 Danny Thomas Place, MS 735, Memphis, TN 38105-3678, USA
* Corresponding author.
E-mail address: wassim.chemaitilly@stjude.org

Endocrinol Metab Clin N Am 41 (2012) 785–792
http://dx.doi.org/10.1016/j.ecl.2012.07.002
0889-8529/12/$ – see front matter © 2012 Elsevier Inc. All rights reserved.

endo.theclinics.com

children with GHD.[2,3] Proved benefits in body composition, bone health, and metabolism have extended the indications for GH replacement to adults with GHD over the past decade.[4,5]

Given the mitogenic and proliferative properties of GH and IGF-1, through hepatic secretion stimulated by GH, the potential association between GH replacement therapy and increased long-term risk of developing a malignancy has been the subject of many reports and reviews.[6–9] Associations between treatment with human-derived pituitary GH and an increased risk of de novo leukemia,[10] cancer-related mortality, and colon cancer[11] have been reported, but none of these findings was subsequently confirmed by studies of patients treated with modern regimens using recombinant (DNA-derived) GH.[12,13] Concerns regarding the long-term safety of GH therapy were reignited by a recent report of higher mortality rates in individuals treated with GH during childhood for idiopathic GHD and non-GHD indications compared with the general population.[14] Although the report, compiling data on 6928 children treated with GH between 1985 and 1996, did not show an increase in cancer-related mortality in this population, there was an increase in mortality related to "bone tumors" (standardized mortality ratio 5.00; CI, 1.01–14.63).[14] Despite the lack of compelling evidence in favor of the association between treatment with recombinant GH and increased cancer risk in the general population of GH-deficient individuals, there are safety concerns among cancer survivors that command additional scrutiny given a proved predisposition for cancer and inherently increased risks of second neoplasms and malignancies.[15,16]

The aim of this review is to discuss available data on the safety of GH replacement therapy in cancer survivors, specifically from the perspective of the potential association between GH replacement and higher cancer recurrence and/or second neoplasm risks. Given that for many years GH was exclusively prescribed in children to promote linear growth, the focus is primarily on childhood cancer survivors.

GROWTH HORMONE, IGF-1, AND CANCER RISK

The IGF system includes 3 growth factors: insulin, IGF-1, and IGF-3; 2 receptors: the insulin receptor, which mediates insulin actions, and the IGF-1 receptor (IGF-1R), which mediates the actions of both IGF-1 and IGF-2; and 6 IGF-binding proteins (IGFBPs) with high binding affinity to the IGFs and low binding affinity to insulin. GH is the main systemic stimulus for the hepatic secretion of circulating endocrine IGF-1. GH also stimulates the secretion of IGFBP-3, which, in turn, regulates the action of IGF-1 through the formation of a stable complex that limits the interaction with IGF-1R.[17] Autocrine/paracrine production of GH and IGF-1 also occur at the level of peripheral tissues. Cellular overexpression of GH and GH receptor and changes in the paracrine/autocrine IGF-1–IGF-1R–IGFBP-3 axis were shown to affect cell cycle and to influence tumor growth in different experimental models.

GH overexpression has been shown to increase in vitro proliferation of both normal and cancerous mammary cells, likely in an autocrine fashion and independently from IGF-1.[9] IGF-1 has mitogenic, proangeiogenic, and antiapoptotic properties, hence promoting tumoral cell growth in several in vitro models.[6–9,17] In contrast, IGFBP-3 seems to exert an inhibitory effect on cancer cell growth and to possess proapoptotic properties that limit tumoral expansion.[6–9,17] Transgenic animal models have provided further corroboration of these properties with situations of tissue-targeted GH or IGF-1 overexpression, leading to higher risks of tumor development, tumor progression, and metastasis. Conversely, tumor growth is inhibited or reversed in models with tissue targeted inhibition of GH and IGF-1 and in models with targeted overexpression of IGFBPs, as summarized in the review by Clayton and colleagues.[6]

The association between cancer risk and increased systemic, endocrine secretion of GH and IGF-1 was mainly studied using 2 approaches: (1) assessment of cancer risk in individuals with acromegaly and (2) measurements of the IGF-1 and IGFBP-3 plasma levels in individuals with different malignancies. There are multiple reports of increased cancer risk in individuals with acromegaly, the more compelling findings related to higher risks of colon cancer, colonic neoplasia, and thyroid cancer.[6] In the general population, weak associations were reported between elevated plasma levels of IGF-1 and increased risks of breast, prostate, and colorectal cancers in several prospective epidemiologic studies.[6,18] These associations do, however, reinforce the need for careful monitoring of IGF-1 levels during GH replacement therapy and bring to attention the particular situation of individuals with GHD who also belong to high-risk groups, such as cancer survivors.[19]

LONG-TERM SAFETY OF GH REPLACEMENT IN CHILDHOOD CANCER SURVIVORS

Childhood cancer survivors are at a significantly higher risk of developing multiple subsequent neoplasms during the course of their lifetime. In a report from the Childhood Cancer Survivor Study (CCSS), a multicenter retrospective cohort of more than 14,000 individuals recruited among 26 institutions in North America, Armstrong and colleagues[16] showed that 9.3% of enrolled subjects (1382 survivors out of 14,358) had developed a second neoplasm. Second neoplasms included, by order of frequency, nonmelanoma skin cancer, breast neoplasms, meningiomas, thyroid cancer, soft tissue sarcomas, and central nervous system malignancies. Even more strikingly, among individuals who had developed second neoplasms, 27.9% went on to further develop additional new neoplasms over the following 20 years.[16] Considering the young age of patients followed in this cohort (the median age at the time of the study was 32 years), genetic predisposition and therapy-related tissue injuries are likely to significantly increase the risk of subsequent tumors and malignancies. Multiple studies have attempted to investigate whether past treatment with GH further increases this risk, including 2 reports from the CCSS.

Treatment with GH and Cancer Recurrence

Several studies concur on the lack of significant association between past treatment with GH and recurrence of the same primary cancer. Reporting on the cumulative incidence of leukemia relapse and second malignancies in 910 survivors of childhood acute lymphoblastic leukemia (ALL), including 47 treated with GH replacement, Leung and colleagues[20] did not find significant differences between GH and non–GH-treated patients after 7 and 11 years of follow-up. In a report on 31 patients treated with GH (24 childhood brain tumor survivors and 7 leukemia survivors exposed to cranial radiotherapy), Clayton and colleagues[21] did not find relapse rates that significantly differed from those observed in non–GH-treated patients. Similar findings were reported in survivors of childhood brain tumors by several consecutive studies.[22] In a report on 207 children treated for various brain tumors, including 47 treated with GH, Ogilvy-Stuart and colleagues[23] did not identify an increased risk of recurrence in children treated with GH (relative risk [RR] 1.01; 95% CI, 0.36–2.83). In a multicenter study of 1071 children diagnosed with brain tumors (patients with craniopharyngioma were not included in this study), including 108 treated with GH, Swerdlow and colleagues[24] also reported that past treatment with GH did not increase the risk of tumor recurrence (RR 0.7; 95% CI, 0.5–1.1). Data collected from large postmarketing surveillance registries, such as Pfizer International Growth Database (KIGS) and the National Cooperative Growth Study (NCGS), with, respectively, more than 50,000 and 19,000 individuals treated with GH, were not suggestive of a higher risk of tumor or cancer recurrence. These studies were limited, however, by lack of non–GH-treated comparison groups.[25,26] In the KIGS registry report, Darendeliler and colleagues[25] compared the observed frequency of tumor recurrence by tumor type to available data in the literature. In patients treated with GH, recurrence rates were 9.8% in individuals with glial tumors (n = 400), 8.8% in those with ependymoma (n = 113), 4.4% in individuals with medulloblastoma (n = 655), and 4.0% in individuals with germinoma (n = 297). These numbers were reported as reassuring when compared with data available on non–GH-treated individuals in other studies, referring in particular to the article by Swerdlow and colleagues.[24,25] In the NCGS report, Blethen and colleagues[26] reported recurrence rates of 7.2% in GH-treated individuals with primitive neuroectodermal tumors (n = 194) and 18.1% in those with low-grade glioma (n = 194). These rates were described as not "excessive" but no further comparisons were provided in the report. In the first CCSS report on the risk of disease recurrence and second neoplasms, Sklar and colleagues[27] did not find a significantly increased risk of cancer recurrence in individuals treated with GH when compared with non–GH-treated survivors. They reported an RR of disease recurrence of 0.83 (95% CI, 0.37–1.86) in individuals treated with GH (n = 361) among 13,539 survivors enrolled in the CCSS at the time.[27] In a more recent single-center retrospective study of 110 survivors of childhood (n = 41) and adult (n = 69) cancer treated with cranial radiotherapy and 110 matched non–GH-treated controls (individuals were matched for radiotherapy dose, age at primary diagnosis, and duration of follow-up), Mackenzie and colleagues[28] did not find significant differences in recurrence rates between the comparison groups (5.5% in the GH-treated group vs 7.3% in controls, P = .78).

Treatment with GH and Second Neoplasms

The initial report from the CCSS by Sklar and colleagues[27] identified an increased risk of second neoplasms in childhood cancer survivors treated with GH when compared with those not treated with GH. In this cohort of 13,222 participants, including 354 patients treated with GH, data regarding second neoplasm occurrence were available. Among individuals treated with GH, 15 developed second neoplasms, including 7 while on GH. All observed second neoplasms in GH-treated individuals were solid tumors and all except 1 involved sites exposed to external radiation. Second neoplasms diagnoses included meningioma (n = 6), osteosarcoma (n = 3), soft tissue sarcoma (n = 2), brain astrocytoma (n = 1), brain glioma (n = 1), mucoepidermoid carcinoma of the parotid (n = 1), and adenocarcinoma of the colon (n = 1). Among survivors not treated with GH, 344 developed second neoplasms. After adjustment for confounding factors, including age at diagnosis, gender, radiation, and alkylating agent effects, exposure to GH significantly increased the risk of second neoplasms (RR 3.21; 95% CI, 1.88–5.46, P<.0001). There was a relative excess of individuals with a primary diagnosis of ALL among GH-treated survivors who developed second neoplasms. When the analysis was restricted to malignant second neoplasms only, treatment with GH was no longer associated with higher risks of second neoplasms. Treatment with GH was not associated with an increased risk of death in this study.[27]

As accrual within the CCSS continued and additional long-term follow-up data became available, an updated report, specifically on the risk of second neoplasms and treatment with GH, was published 4 years later.[29] The expanded CCSS cohort included 14,108 childhood cancer survivors, 361 treated with GH. The findings reported by Ergun-Longmire and colleagues[29] continued to demonstrate that treatment with GH was associated with an increased risk of second neoplasms. The investigators reported 20 cases of second neoplasms in survivors treated with GH, all solid tumors. Diagnoses included meningioma (n = 9), osteosarcoma (n = 3), soft tissue sarcoma (n = 2), brain glioma (n = 2), brain astrocytoma (n = 1), papillary thyroid carcinoma (n = 1), mucoepidermoid carcinoma of parotid (n = 1), and colon adenocarcinoma (n = 1). Among survivors not treated with GH, 555 developed second neoplasms. After adjustment for confounding factors, including age at diagnosis, gender, radiation, and alkylating agent effects, treatment with GH remained independently associated with a higher risk of developing a second neoplasm, although the magnitude of the risk was somewhat lower than the initial analysis (RR 2.15; 95% CI, 1.33–3.47; P = .002). When results were stratified by the initial diagnosis of cancer, no diagnostic category seemed associated with a higher risk of developing second neoplasms. The updated report included data on GH dose and duration of therapy and neither was associated with the risk of developing a second neoplasm. Meningioma was the most common diagnosis among second neoplasms observed in individuals treated with GH; all individuals who developed it were exposed to cranial radiotherapy, itself a known risk factor for meningioma.[30] The latency period for developing a meningioma was shorter in individuals treated with GH than in those who developed meningiomas but were not treated with GH (n = 62), 12.2 years versus 19 years (P<.01). Treatment with GH was not associated with an increased risk of death in this study.[29]

The CCSS reports on the risk of second neoplasms in childhood cancer survivors treated with GH had a lasting impact on clinical practice and patient counseling. The decrease in the RR with longer follow-up and the possibility of ascertainment bias related to a closer monitoring of individuals treated with GH have nevertheless led some investigators to question the findings in these reports.[28] In a recent article by Mackenzie and colleagues[28] on 110 survivors of childhood and adult cancer treated with cranial radiotherapy and 110 matched non–GH-treated controls and followed in a single institution for a median of 14.5 years, individuals treated with GH did not have a higher risk of developing second neoplasms than those not treated with GH. In this study, 5 individuals treated with GH developed second neoplasms (4 meningioma and 1 malignant nerve sheath tumor) versus 3 individuals not treated with GH (2 meningioma and 1 oligodendroglioma). Individuals were matched for radiotherapy dose, age at primary diagnosis, and duration of follow-up. The mean latency period for the diagnosis of meningioma in this cohort was 22.5 ± 6.3 years and was not found to differ significantly between individuals treated with GH and others. When considering the 41 matched pairs for childhood cancer survivors, 5 secondary tumors occurred among survivors versus 2 among the controls (a 2.5-fold difference). This is similar to the magnitude of difference reported by the CCSS.[29]

SAFETY OF ADULT GH REPLACEMENT REGIMENS IN SURVIVORS OF CANCER

With the recent expansion of GH replacement therapy indications to adults with GHD, specific data on the long-term safety of this therapy when administered to adult cancer survivors remain scarce. In an article on the neuroimaging surveillance of 45 brain tumor survivors treated with adult GH replacement therapy over a period of 6.7 ± 3.6 years, Jostel and colleagues[31] reported detecting the appearance of second neoplasms in 5 individuals (all were meningioma cases) during the course of therapy. The investigators also reported observing the progression of meningiomas detected before GH replacement therapy (n = 4) and of one residual primary tumor. Meningiomas occurred on average 22.8 years after exposure to cranial radiotherapy and although they did not relate an increased risk of brain tumor recurrence due to GH therapy, the investigators recommended a systematic neuroimaging surveillance of such individuals, including baseline scans before the initiation of GH replacement and repeat studies at least once after 12 to 18 months of treatment.[31] With the primary aim of reporting on the risk of primary cancers in GH-treated adult hypopituitary patients by analyzing a cohort of 6840 GH-treated and 940 non–GH-treated individuals and by using expected case count reference data for standardized incidence ratio (SIR) calculations, Child and colleagues[32] provide some information on the occurrence of second malignancies on a subset of individuals with a previous diagnosis of cancer who were enrolled in their study. The mean follow-up duration in this study was 3.7 years per GH-treated patient. In total, 138 patients treated as adults with GH developed a cancer versus 32 non–GH-treated individuals. Although the study did not show an overall higher risk of developing a de novo cancer in individuals treated with GH in both the general (SIR 0.88; 95% CI, 0.74–1.04) and United States (SIR 0.94; 95% CI, 0.73–1.18) cohorts, there was a higher than expected incidence of newly diagnosed cancers in individuals 35 years and younger enrolled in the United States cohort (SIR 3.79; CI, 1.39–8.26) based on 6 observed cancers versus an expected reference count of 1.58. The investigators noted that 5 of these 6 patients had a previously diagnosed malignancy (this was a second cancer) and 4 of 6 individuals had childhood-onset GHD. These observations reflect the known relative vulnerability of childhood cancer survivors to second cancers[16] when compared with individuals with similar ages in the general population and call for continued caution in their risk assessment.

SUMMARY

Treatment with GH replacement does not seem to increase the risk of disease recurrence and mortality in survivors of childhood cancers. An increased risk of second neoplasms has been reported in survivors treated with GH when compared with those not receiving GH replacement. This risk seems to involve primarily a higher incidence of meningiomas in GH-replaced individuals who were treated with cranial radiotherapy. It remains unclear what the true magnitude of risk may be for GH exposure given the small sample sizes and potential for residual confounding by radiation therapy exposure. Longer-term follow-up is necessary to confirm if this higher RR persists or changes over time. The expansion of GH indications beyond the years of childhood has brought about the need for close monitoring and prospective safety data, especially in childhood cancer survivors, given their known higher risks for subsequent neoplasms and long-term health concerns.

REFERENCES

1. Chemaitilly W, Sklar CA. Endocrine complications in long-term survivors of childhood cancers. Endocr Relat Cancer 2010;17:R141–59.
2. Adan L, Sainte-Rose C, Souberbielle JC, et al. Adult height after growth hormone (GH) treatment for GH deficiency due to cranial irradiation. Med Pediatr Oncol 2000;34:14–9.
3. Gleeson HK, Stoeter R, Ogilvy-Stuart AL, et al. Improvements in final height over 25 years in growth hormone (GH)-deficient childhood survivors of brain tumours receiving GH replacement. J Clin Endocrinol Metab 2003;88:3682–9.
4. Mukherjee A, Tolhurst-Cleaver S, Ryder WD, et al. The characteristics of quality of life impairment in adult growth hormone (GH)-deficient survivors of cancer and their response to GH replacement therapy. J Clin Endocrinol Metab 2005;90:1542–9.
5. Murray RD, Darzy KH, Gleeson HK, et al. GH deficient survivors of childhood cancer: GH replacement during adult life. J Clin Endocrinol Metab 2002;87:129–35.

6. Clayton PE, Banerjee I, Murray PG, et al. Growth hormone, the insulin-like growth factor axis, insulin and cancer risk. Nat Rev Endocrinol 2011;7:11–24.
7. Jenkins PJ, Mukherjee A, Shalet SM. Does growth hormone cause cancer? Clin Endocrinol 2006;64:115–21.
8. Ogilvy-Stuart AL, Gleeson H. Cancer risk following growth hormone use in childhood. Implications for current practice. Drug Saf 2004;27:369–82.
9. Cohen P, Clemmons DR, Rosenfeld RG. Does the GH-IGF axis play a role in cancer pathogenesis? Growth Horm IGF Res 2000;10:297–305.
10. Fradkin JE, Mills JL, Schonberger LB, et al. Risk of leukemia after treatment with pituitary growth hormone. JAMA 1993;270:2829–32.
11. Swerdlow AJ, Higgins CD, Adlard P, et al. Risk of cancer in patients treated with human pituitary growth horone in the UK, 1959-85: a cohort study. Lancet 2002; 360:273–7.
12. Allen DB, Chen Rundle A, Graves DA, et al. Risk of leukemia in children treated with human growth horone: review and reanalysis. J Pediatr 1997;131:S32–6.
13. Tuffli GA, Johanson A, Chen Rundle A, et al. Lack of increased risk for extracranial, non leukemic neoplasms in recipients of recombinant deoxyribonucleic acid growth hormone. J Clin Endocrinol Metab 1995;80:1416–22.
14. Carel JC, Ecosse E, Landier F, et al. Long-term mortality after recombinant growth hormone treatment for isolated growth hormone deficiency or childhood short stature: preliminary report on the French SAGhE study. J Clin Endocrinol Metab 2012;97:416–25.
15. Neglia JP, Friedman DL, Yasui Y, et al. Second malignant neoplasms in five-year survivors of childhood cancer: childhood cancer survivor study. J Natl Cancer Inst 2001;93:618–29.
16. Armstrong GT, Liu W, Leisenring W, et al. Occurrence of multiple subsequent neoplasms in long-term survivors of childhood cancer: a report from the childhood cancer survivor study. J Clin Oncol 2011;29:3056–64.
17. LeRoith D, Butler AA. Insulin-like growth factors in pediatric health and disease. J Clin Endocrinol Metab 1999;84:4355–61.
18. Renehan AG, Zwahlen M, Minder C, et al. Insulin-like growth factor (IGF)-I, IGF binding protein-3 and cancer risk: systematic review and meta-regression analysis. Lancet 2004;363:1346–53.
19. Rosenfeld RG, Cohen P, Robison LL, et al. Long-term surveillance of growth hormone therapy. J Clin Endocrinol Metab 2012;97:68–72.
20. Leung W, Rose SR, Zhou Y, et al. Outcomes of growth hormone replacement therapy in survivors of childhood acute lymphoblastic leukemia. J Clin Oncol 2002;13:2959–64.
21. Clayton PE, Shalet SM, Gattamaneni HR, et al. Does growth hormone cause relapse of brain tumours? Lancet 1987;1(8535):711–3.
22. Bogarin R, Steinbok P. Growth hormone treatment and risk of recurrence or progression of brain tumors in children: a review. Childs Nerv Syst 2009;25: 273–9.
23. Ogilvy-Stuart AL, Ryder WDJ, Gattamaneni HR, et al. Growth hormone and tumour recurrence. BMJ 1992;304:1601–5.
24. Swerdlow AJ, Reddingius RE, Higgins CD, et al. Growth hormone treatment of children with brain tumors and risk of tumor recurrence. J Clin Endocrinol Metab 2000;85:4444–9.
25. Darendeliler F, Karagiannis G, Wilton P, et al. Recurrence of brain tumours in patients treated with growth hormone: analysis of KIGS (Pfizer International Growth Database). Acta Paediatr 2006;95:1284–90.

26. Blethen SL, Allen DB, Graves D, et al. Safety of recombinant deoxyribonucleic acid derived growth hormone: the National Cooperative Growth Study experience. J Clin Endocrinol Metab 1996;81:1704–10.

27. Sklar CA, Mertens AC, Mitby P, et al. Risk of disease recurrence and second neoplasms in survivors of childhood cancer treated with growth hormone: a report from the childhood cancer survivor study. J Clin Endocrinol Metab 2002;87: 3136–41.

28. Mackenzie S, Craven T, Gattamaneni HR, et al. Long-term safety of growth hormone replacement after CNS irradiation. J Clin Endocrinol Metab 2011;96: 2756–61.

29. Ergun-Longmire B, Mertens AC, Mitby P, et al. Growth hormone and risk of second neoplasms in the childhood cancer survivor study. J Clin Endocrinol Metab 2006;91:3494–8.

30. Paulino AC, Ahmed IM, Mai WY, et al. The influence of pretreatment characteristics and radiotherapy parameters on time interval to development of radiation-associated meningioma. Int J Radiat Oncol Biol Phys 2009;75:1408–14.

31. Jostel A, Mukherjee A, Hulse PA, et al. Adult growth hormone replacement therapy and neuroimaging surveillance in brain tumour survivors. Clin Endocrinol 2005;62:698–705.

32. Child CJ, Zimmermann AG, Woodmansee WW, et al. Assessment of primary cancers in GH-treated adult hypopituitary patients: an analysis from the hypopituitary control and complications study. Eur J Endocrinol 2011;165:217–23.

Cushing Syndrome in Pediatrics

Constantine A. Stratakis, MD, D (Med) Sci[a,b,*]

KEYWORDS

- Cushing syndrome • Pituitary tumors • Cortisol • Adrenal cortex • Carney complex
- Adrenocortical hyperplasia • Adrenal cancer

KEY POINTS

- Cushing syndrome in childhood results mostly from the exogenous administration of glucocorticoids; endogenous Cushing syndrome is a rare disease.
- Barriers to optimal care of a pediatric patient with Cushing syndrome are: improper following of the proper sequence of testing for diagnosing this disease, which stems from lack of understanding of pathophysiology of the hypothalamic-pituitary-adrenal axis; lack of access to proper (ie, experienced, state-of-the-art) surgical treatment; and unavailability of well-tolerated and effective medications to control hypercortisolemia.

Corticotropin (ACTH)-releasing hormone (CRH) is synthesized in the hypothalamus and carried to the anterior pituitary in the portal system. CRH stimulates ACTH release from the anterior pituitary, which in turn stimulates the adrenal cortex to secrete cortisol (hypothalamic-pituitary-adrenal or HPA axis).[1–4] Cortisol inhibits the synthesis and secretion of both CRH and ACTH in a negative feedback regulation system. In Cushing syndrome, the HPA axis has lost its ability for self-regulation, due to excessive secretion of either ACTH or cortisol and the loss of the negative feedback function. Diagnostic tests, on the other hand, take advantage of the tight regulation of the HPA axis in the normal state and its disturbance in Cushing syndrome to guide therapy toward the primary cause of this disorder.

This work was completed with support by the Intramural Program of the Eunice Kennedy Shriver National Institute of Child Health and Human Development, National Institutes of Health, Bethesda, MD 20892–1862.

The author has nothing to disclose.

a Section on Endocrinology and Genetics, Program in Developmental Endocrinology and Genetics, *Eunice Kennedy Shriver* National Institute of Child Health and Human Development, National Institutes of Health, Bethesda, MD 20892–1862, USA; b Pediatric Endocrinology Training Program, National Institute of Child Health and Human Development, National Institutes of Health, Building 10, CRC, Room 1–3330 East Laboratories, 10 Center Drive, Bethesda, MD 20892, USA

* Pediatric Endocrinology Training Program, National Institute of Child Health and Human Development, National Institutes of Health, Building 10, CRC, Room 1–3330 East Laboratories, 10 Center Drive, Bethesda, MD 20892.

E-mail address: stratakc@mail.nih.gov

Endocrinol Metab Clin N Am 41 (2012) 793–803
http://dx.doi.org/10.1016/j.ecl.2012.08.002
0889-8529/12/$ – see front matter Published by Elsevier Inc.

endo.theclinics.com

EPIDEMIOLOGY AND ETIOLOGY

Cushing syndrome is a rare entity, especially in children.[1] The overall incidence of Cushing syndrome is approximately 2 to 5 new cases per million people per year. Only approximately 10% of the new cases each year occur in children. As in adult patients, in children with Cushing syndrome there is a female-to-male predominance, which decreases with younger age. There might even be a male-to-female predominance in infants and young toddlers with Cushing syndrome.[1,3,4] The most common cause of Cushing syndrome in children is exogenous or iatrogenic Cushing syndrome. This is the result of chronic administration of glucocorticoids or ACTH. Glucocorticoids are being used more frequently for the treatment of many nonendocrine diseases including pulmonary, autoimmune, dermatologic, hematologic, and neoplastic disorders. In addition, ACTH is being used for the treatment of certain seizure disorders. The most common cause of endogenous Cushing syndrome in children is ACTH overproduction from the pituitary called Cushing disease. It is usually caused by an ACTH-secreting pituitary microadenoma and, rarely, a macroadenoma. ACTH secretion occurs in a semiautonomous manner, maintaining some of the feedback of the HPA axis. Cushing disease accounts for approximately 75% of all cases of Cushing syndrome in children over 7 years. In children under 7 years, Cushing disease is less frequent; adrenal causes of Cushing syndrome (adenoma, carcinoma, or bilateral hyperplasia) are the most common causes of the condition in infants and young toddlers. Ectopic ACTH production occurs rarely in young children; it also accounts for less than 1% of the cases of Cushing syndrome in adolescents. Sources of ectopic ACTH include small cell carcinoma of the lung, carcinoid tumors in the bronchus, pancreas, or thymus; medullary carcinomas of the thyroid, pheochromocytomas; and other neuroendocrine tumors, especially those of the pancreas and gut carcinoids. Rarely, ACTH overproduction by the pituitary may be the result of CRH oversecretion by the hypothalamus or by an ectopic CRH source. However, this cause of Cushing syndrome has only been described in a small number of cases, and never in young children. Its significance lies in the fact that diagnostic tests that are usually used for the exclusion of ectopic sources of Cushing syndrome have frequently misleading results in the case of CRH-induced ACTH oversecretion. Autonomous secretion of cortisol from the adrenal glands, or ACTH-independent Cushing syndrome, accounts for approximately 15% of all the cases of Cushing syndrome in childhood. However, although adrenocortical tumors are rare in older children, in younger children they are more frequent. In prepubertal children, adrenocortical lesions are the most frequent cause of Cushing syndrome. Adrenocortical neoplasms account for 0.6% of all childhood tumors; Cushing syndrome is a manifestation of approximately one-third of all adrenal tumors.[3–5] In young children, unilateral (single) adrenal tumors presenting with Cushing syndrome are often malignant (more than 70%). Most patients present under age 5, contributing thus to the first peak of the known bimodal distribution of adrenal cancer across the life span. As in adults, there is a female-to-male predominance. The tumors usually occur unilaterally; however, in 2% to 10% of patients they occur bilaterally. Recently, bilateral nodular adrenal disease has been appreciated as a more frequent than previously thought cause of Cushing syndrome in childhood.[5,6] Primary pigmented adrenocortical nodular disease (PPNAD) is a genetic disorder with the majority of cases associated with Carney complex, a syndrome of multiple endocrine gland abnormalities in addition to lentigines and myxomas. The adrenal glands in PPNAD are most commonly normal or even small in size, with multiple pigmented nodules usually (but not always) surrounded by an atrophic cortex. The nodules are autonomously functioning, resulting in the surrounding atrophy of the cortex. Children and adolescents with PPNAD frequently have periodic, cyclical, or otherwise atypical Cushing syndrome. Massive macronodular adrenal hyperplasia (MMAD) is another rare bilateral disease that leads to Cushing syndrome.[5] The adrenal glands are massively enlarged, with multiple, huge nodules that are typical yellow-to-brown cortisol-producing adenomas. Most cases of MMAD are sporadic, although a few familial cases have been described; in those cases, the disease appears in children. In some patients with MMAD, cortisol levels appear to increase with food ingestion (food-dependent Cushing syndrome). These patients have an aberrant expression of the gastric inhibitory polypeptide receptor (GIPR) in the adrenal glands. In the majority of patients with MMAD, however, the disease does not appear to be GIPR-dependent; aberrant expression of other receptors may be responsible for the disease in these patients. Adrenal adenomas or, more frequently, bilateral macronodular adrenal hyperplasia can also be seen in McCune Albright syndrome (MAS).[7,8] In this syndrome, there is a somatic mutation of the *GNAS1* gene leading to constitutive activation of the Gsα protein and continuous, non-ACTH-dependent activation of steroidogenesis by the adrenal cortex. Cushing syndrome in MAS is rare and usually presents in the infantile period (before 6 months of age); interestingly, a few children have had spontaneous resolution of their Cushing syndrome. Aberrant cyclic adenosine monophosphate (cAMP) signaling has been linked to almost all genetic forms of adrenal-dependent cortisol excess. PPNAD is associated with germline inactivating mutations of the *PRKAR1A* gene.[9] Several other forms of micronodular bilateral adrenocortical hyperplasia (BAH) are not associated with inactivating mutations of the *PRKAR1A* gene, but may occur as de novo or autosomal-dominant inheritance of mutations, in the *PDE11A* or *PDE8B* genes.[10,11] Among functional pituitary tumors in early childhood, ACTH-producing adenomas are probably the most common, although they are still considerably rare. To date, no genetic defects have been consistently associated with childhood corticotropinomas, which only rarely occur in the familial setting, and then, most commonly in the context of multiple endocrine neoplasia type 1 (MEN 1) and rarely due to *AIP* mutations.[12,13]

CLINICAL PRESENTATION

In most children, the onset of Cushing syndrome is insidious.[1,3,4,14] The most common presenting symptom is weight gain; in childhood, lack of height gain consistent with the weight gain is the most common presentation of Cushing syndrome. A typical growth chart for a child with Cushing syndrome is shown in **Fig. 1**. Other common problems reported in children include facial plethora, headaches, hypertension, hirsutism, amenorrhea, and delayed sexual development. Pubertal children may present with virilization. Skin manifestations, including acne, violaceous striae, bruising, and acanthosis nigricans are also common.[2] Compared with adult patients with Cushing syndrome, symptoms that are less commonly seen in children include sleep disruption, muscular weakness, and problems with memory.

DIAGNOSTIC GUIDELINES

The appropriate therapeutic interventions in Cushing syndrome depend on accurate diagnosis and classification of the disease. The medical history and clinical evaluation, including review of growth data, are important to make the initial diagnosis of Cushing syndrome. Upon suspicion of Cushing syndrome, laboratory and imaging confirmations are necessary. An algorithm of the diagnostic process is presented in **Fig. 2**.

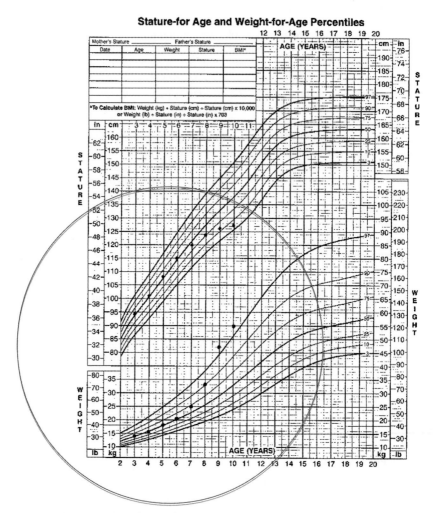

Fig. 1. Typical growth chart for a patient with Cushing syndrome.

The first step in the diagnosis of Cushing syndrome is to document hypercortisolism,[15,16] which is typically done in the outpatient setting. Because of the circadian nature of cortisol and ACTH, isolated cortisol and ACTH measurements are not of great value in diagnosis. One excellent screening test for hypercortisolism is a 24-hour urinary free cortisol (UFC) excretion (corrected for body surface area). However, it is often difficult to obtain a 24-hour urine collection reliably in the outpatient setting, particularly in the pediatric population. Falsely high UFC may be obtained because of physical and emotional stress, chronic and severe obesity, pregnancy, chronic exercise, depression, poor diabetes control, alcoholism, anorexia, narcotic withdrawal, anxiety, malnutrition, and high water intake. These conditions may cause sufficiently high UFCs to cause what is known as pseudo-Cushing syndrome. On the other hand, falsely low UFC may be obtained mostly with inadequate collection.

Another baseline test for the establishment of the diagnosis of Cushing syndrome is a low-dose dexamethasone suppression test. This test involves giving 1 mg of

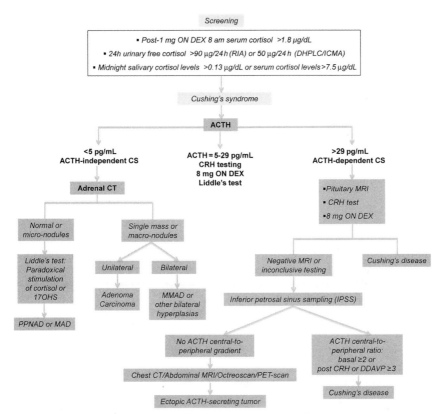

Fig. 2. Diagnostic algorithm in Cushing syndrome.

dexamethasone at 11 and measuring a serum cortisol level the following morning at 8 AM. If the serum cortisol level is greater than 1.8 µg/dL, further evaluation is necessary.[17] This test has a low percentage of false-normal suppression; however, the percentage of false positives is higher (approximately 15% to 20%). It should be remembered that the 1 mg overnight test, like the 24-hour UFCs, does not distinguish between hypercortisolism from Cushing syndrome and other hypercortisolemic states. If the response to the 1 mg dexamethasone overnight suppression test and the 24-hour UFC are both normal, a diagnosis of Cushing syndrome may be excluded with the following caveat: 5% to 10% of patients may have intermittent or periodic cortisol hypersecretion and may not manifest abnormal results to either test. If periodic or intermittent Cushing syndrome is suspected, continuous follow-up of the patients is recommended, including monitoring of growth and 24-hour UFC. If one of the test results is suggestive of Cushing syndrome, or if there is any question about the diagnosis, then tests that distinguish between pseudo-Cushing syndrome states and Cushing syndrome may be obtained. One such test is the combined dexamethasone-CRH test.[18] In this test, the patient is treated with low-dose dexamethasone (0.5 mg adjusted for weight for children <70 kg) every 6 hours for 8 doses before the administration of CRH (ovine CRH-oCRH) the following morning. ACTH and cortisol levels are measured at baseline (-15, -5, and 0 min) and 15 minutes after the administration of oCRH (plasma dexamethasone level is measured once at baseline). The patient with pseudo-Cushing syndrome will exhibit low or undetectable basal plasma cortisol and ACTH and have a diminished or no response to oCRH stimulation.

Patients with Cushing syndrome will have higher basal cortisol and ACTH levels and will also have a greater peak value with oCRH stimulation. A cortisol level of greater than 1.4 μg/dL (38 nmol/L) 15 minutes after oCRH administration supports a diagnosis of Cushing syndrome, and further evaluation is indicated. However, the author and colleagues recently reported that severe obesity (body mass index [BMI] greater than 2 standard deviations [SD]) confounds the interpretation of the dexamethasone-CRH test. Confirmed height gain is a simple way to help distinguish children with pseudo-Cushing from those with Cushing syndrome.[19] Once the diagnosis of Cushing syndrome is confirmed, there are several tests to distinguish ACTH-dependent disease from the ACTH-independent syndrome.

A spot morning plasma ACTH may be measured; we have recently reported that a cutoff value of 29 pg/mL in children with confirmed Cushing syndrome has a sensitivity of 70% in identifying children with an ACTH-dependent form of the syndrome.[15] It is important to consider the variability in plasma ACTH levels and the instability of the molecule after the sample's collection. The standard high-dose dexamethasone suppression test (HDDST or Liddle's test) is used to differentiate Cushing disease from ectopic ACTH secretion and adrenal causes of Cushing syndrome. The Liddle's test has been modified to giving a high dose of dexamethasone (120 μg/kg, maximum dose 8 mg) at 11 PM and measuring the plasma cortisol level the following morning. We have recently reported in a pediatric population that 20% cortisol suppression from baseline had sensitivity and specificity of 97.5% and 100%, respectively, with the HDDST for differentiating patients with Cushing disease from those with adrenal tumors.[15] Indications for obtaining the classic Liddle's test, low-dose dexamethasone (30 μg/kg/dose; maximum 0.5 mg/dose) every 6 hours for 8 doses, followed by high-dose dexamethasone (120 μg/kg/dose; maximum 2 mg/dose) every 6 hours for 8 doses (instead of the modified overnight HDDST), include nonsuppression of serum cortisol levels during the HDDST and/or negative imaging studies, and/or suspected adrenal disease. UFC and 17-hydroxysteroid (17OHS) excretion are measured at baseline and after dexamethasone administration during Liddle's test. Approximately 85% of patients with Cushing disease will have suppression of serum cortisol, UFC, and 17OHS values, whereas less than 10% of patients with ectopic ACTH secretion will have suppression. UFC values should suppress to 90% of baseline value, and 17OHS excretion should suppress to less than 50% of baseline value. This test has been shown to be useful mostly in patients who have suspected adrenal disease; in this case it is used with the aim of identifying a paradoxic stimulation of cortisol secretion, which is found in patients with PPNAD and other forms of BAH, but not in other forms of primary adrenocortical lesions.[20]

We have recently reported in a larger series of pediatric patients that following confirmation of elevated 24-hour UFC (3 collections), a single midnight cortisol value of greater than 4.4 μg/dL followed by a high-dose dexamethasone suppression test (>20% suppression of morning serum cortisol) was the most rapid and accurate way for confirmation and diagnostic differentiation, respectively, of hypercortisolemia due to a pituitary or adrenal tumor.[15] However, for accuracy, diurnal testing requires an inpatient stay, and this may limit its use as a routine screening test.[15] An oCRH stimulation test may also be obtained for the differentiation of Cushing disease from ectopic ACTH secretion[21] and/or adrenal lesions. In this test, 85% of patients with Cushing disease respond to oCRH with increased plasma ACTH and cortisol production. Ninety-five percent of patients with ectopic ACTH production do not respond to administration of oCRH. The criterion for diagnosis of Cushing disease is a mean increase of 20% above baseline for cortisol values at 30 and 45 minutes and an increase in the mean corticotropin concentrations of at least 35% over basal value at 15 and 30 minutes after CRH administration. When the oCRH and high-dose dexamethasone (Liddle's or overnight) tests are used together, diagnostic accuracy improves to 98%. The oCRH test should not be used in patients with atypical forms of Cushing syndrome, because individuals with normal pituitary function respond to oCRH like patients with Cushing disease. Interpretation of oCRH testing in the differential diagnosis of Cushing syndrome is only possible when the normal corticotrophs are suppressed by consistently elevated cortisol levels.

Another important tool in the localization and characterization of Cushing syndrome is diagnostic imaging. The most important initial imaging when Cushing disease is suspected is pituitary magnetic resonance imaging (MRI). The MRI should be done in thin sections with high resolution and always with contrast (gadolinium). The latter is important, since only macroadenomas will be detectable without contrast; after contrast, an otherwise normal-looking pituitary MRI might show a hypoenhancing lesion, usually a microadenoma. More than 90% of ACTH-producing tumors are hypoenhancing, whereas only about 5% are hyperenhancing after contrast infusion. However, even with the use of contrast material, pituitary MRI may detect only up to approximately 50% of ACTH-producing pituitary tumors. Recently, the author and colleagues reported that postcontrast spoiled gradient-recalled MRI (SPGR-MRI) was superior to spin echo MRI (SE-MRI) in the detection of a microadenoma in children and adolescents with Cushing disease.[22] Computed tomography (CT) (more preferable than MRI) of the adrenal glands is useful in the distinction between Cushing disease and adrenal causes of Cushing syndrome, mainly unilateral adrenal tumors. The distinction is harder in the presence of bilateral hyperplasia (MMAD or PPNAD) or the rare case of bilateral adrenal carcinoma. Most patients with Cushing disease have ACTH-driven bilateral hyperplasia, and both adrenal glands will appear enlarged and nodular on CT or MRI. Most adrenocortical carcinomas are unilateral and quite large by the time they are detected. Adrenocortical adenomas are usually small, less than 5 cm in diameter, and, like most carcinomas, they involve 1 adrenal gland. MMAD presents with massive enlargement of both adrenal glands, whereas PPNAD is more difficult to diagnose radiologically, because it is usually associated with normal- or small-sized adrenal glands, despite the histologic presence of hyperplasia. A CT or MRI scan of the neck, chest, abdomen, and pelvis may be used for the detection of an ectopic source of ACTH production. Labeled octreotide scanning, positron-emission tomography (PET), and venous sampling may also help in the localization of an ectopic ACTH source.

Since up to 50% of pituitary ACTH-secreting tumors and many of ectopic ACTH tumors may not be detected on routine imaging, and often laboratory diagnosis is not completely clear, catheterization studies must be used to confirm the source of ACTH secretion in ACTH-dependent Cushing syndrome. Bilateral inferior petrosal sinus sampling (IPSS) has been used for the localization of a pituitary microadenoma[23]; however, we have recently reported that it is a poor predictor of the site of a microadenoma in children.[24] In brief, sampling from each inferior petrosal sinus is taken for measurement of ACTH concentration simultaneously with peripheral venous sampling. ACTH is measured at baseline and at 3, 5, and 10 minutes after oCRH administration. Patients with ectopic ACTH secretion have no gradient between either sinus (central) and the peripheral sample. On the other hand, patients with an ACTH-secreting pituitary adenoma have at least a 2-to-1 central-to-peripheral gradient at baseline or 3-to-1 central-to-peripheral gradient after stimulation with oCRH. IPSS is an excellent test for the differential diagnosis between ACTH-dependent forms of Cushing syndrome with a diagnostic accuracy that approximates 100%, as long as it is performed in an experienced clinical center. IPSS, however, may not lead to the correct diagnosis if it is obtained when the patient is not sufficiently hypercortisolemic or if venous drainage of the pituitary gland does not follow the expected, normal anatomy, or with an ectopic CRH-producing tumor.

TREATMENT

The treatment of choice for almost all patients with an ACTH-secreting pituitary adenoma (Cushing disease) is transsphenoidal surgery (TSS). In most specialized centers with experienced neurosurgeons, the success rate of the first TSS is 90%[25] or higher. Treatment failures are most commonly the result of a macroadenoma or a small tumor invading the cavernous sinus. The success rate of repeat TSS is lower, closer to 60%. Postoperative complications include transient diabetes insipidus (DI) and, occasionally, syndrome of inappropriate antidiuretic hormone secretion (SIADH), central hypothyroidism, growth hormone deficiency, hypogonadism, bleeding, infection (meningitis), and pituitary apoplexy. The mortality rate is extremely low, at less than 1%. Permanent pituitary dysfunction (partial or pan-hypopituitarism) and DI are rare but they are more likely after repeat TSS or larger adenomas. Pituitary irradiation is considered an appropriate treatment in patients with Cushing disease following a failed TSS. Up to 80% of patients will have remission after irradiation of the pituitary gland. Hypopituitarism is the most common adverse effect, and it is more frequent when surgery precedes the radiotherapy. The recommended dosage is 4500/5000 cGy total, usually given over a period of 6 weeks. Newer forms of stereotactic radiotherapy are now available as options for treatment of ACTH-secreting pituitary tumors. Photon knife (computer-assisted linear accelerator) or the gamma knife (cobalt –60) approaches are now available; however, experience with these techniques is limited, especially in children. These modalities may be attractive because of the smaller amount of time required for these procedures and the possibility for fewer adverse effects.

The treatment of choice for benign adrenal tumors is surgical resection. This procedure can be done by either transperitoneal or retroperitoneal approaches. In addition, laparoscopic adrenalectomy is also available at many institutions. Adrenal carcinomas may also be surgically resected, unless at later stages. Solitary metastases should be removed, if possible.[26] Therapy with mitotane, which is an adrenocytolytic agent, can be used as an adjuvant therapy or in the case of an inoperable tumor. Other chemotherapeutic options include cisplatin, 5-flourouracil, suramin, doxorubicin, and etoposide. Occasionally glucocorticoid antagonists and steroid synthesis inhibitors are needed to correct the hypercortisolism. Radiotherapy can also be used in the case of metastases. The prognosis for adrenal carcinoma is poor, but usually children have a better prognosis than adults.

Bilateral total adrenalectomy is usually the treatment of choice in bilateral micronodular or macronodular adrenal disease, such as PPNAD and MMAD. In addition, adrenalectomy may be considered as a treatment for those patients with Cushing disease or ectopic ACTH-dependent Cushing syndrome who have either failed surgery or radiotherapy, or their tumor has not been localized, respectively. Nelson syndrome, which includes increased pigmentation, elevated ACTH levels, and a growing pituitary ACTH-producing pituitary tumor, may develop in up to 15% of patients with Cushing disease who are treated with bilateral adrenalectomy. It is possible that children with untreated Cushing disease are especially vulnerable to Nelson syndrome after bilateral adrenalectomy.

Pharmacotherapy is an option in the case of failure of surgery for Cushing disease or in ectopic ACTH secretion where the source cannot be identified. Mitotane inhibits the biosynthesis of corticosteroids by blocking the action of 11-β-hydroxylase and cholesterol side chain cleavage enzymes. It also acts by destroying adrenocortical cells that secrete cortisol. Other adrenal enzyme inhibitors, such as aminoglutethimide, metyrapone, trilostane, and ketoconazole, may also be used alone or in combinations to control hypercortisolism. Aminoglutethimide blocks the conversion of cholesterol to pregnenolone in the adrenal cortex, inhibiting the synthesis of cortisol, aldosterone, and androgens. Metyrapone acts by preventing the conversion of 11-deoxycortisol to cortisol. It can also cause hypertension secondary to the accumulation of 11-deoxycorticosterone. Trilostane inhibits the conversion of pregnenolone to progesterone. Ketoconazole is an agent that affects many pathway steps and is excellent in blocking adrenal steroidogenesis.

In ectopic ACTH production, if the source of ACTH secretion can be identified, then the treatment of choice is surgical resection of the tumor. If surgical resection is impossible or if the source of ACTH cannot be identified, then pharmacotherapy is indicated as previously discussed. If the tumor cannot be located, then repeat searches for the tumor should be performed at least yearly. Bilateral adrenalectomy should be performed in the case of failure of pharmacotherapy or failure to locate the tumor after many years.

GLUCOCORTICOID REPLACEMENT

After the completion of successful TSS in Cushing disease or excision of an autonomously functioning adrenal adenoma, there will be a period of adrenal insufficiency while the hypothalamic pituitary adrenal axis is recovering. During this period, glucocorticoids should be replaced at the suggested physiologic replacement dose (12–15 mg/m^2/day 2 or 3 times daily), as we have recently published.[27] In the immediate postoperative period, stress doses of cortisol should be initiated. These should be weaned relatively rapidly to a physiologic replacement dose; the patient should be followed every few months, and the adrenocortical function should be periodically assessed with a 1-hour ACTH test (normal response is a cortisol level over 18 ug/dL at 30 or 60 minutes after ACTH stimulation).

Patients after unilateral adrenalectomy for a single adrenocortical tumor, require the same replacement and regimen as patients with cushing disease post-TSS. After bilateral adrenalectomy, patients require lifetime replacement with both glucocorticoids (as described previously) and mineralocorticoids (fludrocortisone 0.1–0.3 mg daily). These patients also need stress doses of glucocorticoids immediately postoperatively; they are weaned to physiologic replacement relatively quickly. In addition, stress dosing for acute illness, trauma, or surgical procedures is required for both temporary and permanent adrenal insufficiency.

PSYCHOSOCIAL IMPLICATIONS

Cushing syndrome has been associated with multiple psychiatric and psychological disturbances, most commonly emotional lability, depression, and/or anxiety. Other abnormalities have included mania, panic disorder, suicidal ideation, schizophrenia, obsessive–compulsive symptomatology, psychosis, impaired self-esteem, and distorted body image. Significant psychopathology can even remain after remission of hypercortisolism and even after recovery of the HPA axis. Up to 70% of patients will have significant improvements in the psychiatric symptoms gradually after the correction of the hypercortisolism. The author and colleagues recently reported that children with Cushing syndrome may experience a decline in cognitive and school performance 1 year after surgical cure, without any associated psychopathology.[28] We recently reported that active Cushing syndrome, particularly in younger children, was associated with low physical and psychosocial scores, and that despite improvement from before to 1 year after cure, residual impairment remained in physical function and role–emotional impact score. Although most self-reported Cushing syndrome symptoms showed improvement, forgetfulness, unclear thinking, and decreased attention span did not improve after cure.[29]

REFERENCES

1. Magiakou MA, Mastorakos G, Oldfield EH, et al. Cushing's syndrome in children and adolescents. Presentation, diagnosis, and therapy. N Engl J Med 1994; 331(10):629–36.
2. Lodish MB, Sinaii N, Patronas N, et al. Blood pressure in pediatric patients with Cushing syndrome. J Clin Endocrinol Metab 2009;94(6):2002–8.
3. Tsigos C, Chrousos GP. Differential diagnosis and management of Cushing's syndrome. Annu Rev Med 1996;47:443–61.
4. Orth DN. Cushing's syndrome. N Engl J Med 1995;332(12):791–803.
5. Stratakis CA, Kirschner LS. Clinical and genetic analysis of primary bilateral adrenal diseases (micro- and macronodular disease) leading to Cushing syndrome. Horm Metab Res 1998;30(6–7):456–63.
6. Stratakis CA. Cushing syndrome caused by adrenocortical tumors and hyperplasias (corticotropin-independent Cushing syndrome). Endocr Dev 2008;13: 117–32.
7. Kirk JM, Brain CE, Carson DJ, et al. Cushing's syndrome caused by nodular adrenal hyperplasia in children with McCune-Albright syndrome. J Pediatr 1999;134(6):789–92.
8. Fragoso MC, Domenice S, Latronico AC, et al. Cushing's syndrome secondary to adrenocorticotropin-independent macronodular adrenocortical hyperplasia due to activating mutations of GNAS1 gene. J Clin Endocrinol Metab 2003;88(5): 2147–51.
9. Kirschner LS, Carney JA, Pack SD, et al. Mutations of the gene encoding the protein kinase a type I-alpha regulatory subunit in patients with the Carney complex. Nat Genet 2000;26(1):89–92.
10. Horvath A, Boikos S, Giatzakis C, et al. A genome-wide scan identifies mutations in the gene encoding phosphodiesterase 11A4 (PDE11A) in individuals with adrenocortical hyperplasia. Nat Genet 2006;38(7):794–800.
11. Gunther DF, Bourdeau I, Matyakhina L, et al. Cyclical Cushing syndrome presenting in infancy: an early form of primary pigmented nodular adrenocortical disease, or a new entity? J Clin Endocrinol Metab 2004;89(7):3173–82.
12. Marx SJ, Agarwal SK, Kester MB, et al. Multiple endocrine neoplasia type 1: clinical and genetic features of the hereditary endocrine neoplasias. Recent Prog Horm Res 1999;54:397–438 [discussion: 438–399].
13. Stratakis CA, Tichomirowa MA, Boikos S, et al. The role of germline *AIP, MEN1, PRKAR1A, CDKN1B* and *CDKN2C* mutations in causing pituitary adenomas in a large cohort of children, adolescents, and patients with genetic syndromes. Clin Genet 2010;78(5):457–63.
14. Magiakou MA, Chrousos GP. Cushing's syndrome in children and adolescents: current diagnostic and therapeutic strategies. J Endocrinol Invest 2002;25(2): 181–94.
15. Batista DL, Riar J, Keil M, et al. Diagnostic tests for children who are referred for the investigation of Cushing syndrome. Pediatrics 2007;120(3):e575–86.

16. Bornstein SR, Stratakis CA, Chrousos GP. Adrenocortical tumors: recent advances in basic concepts and clinical management. Ann Intern Med 1999; 130(9):759–71.
17. Nieman LK, Biller BM, Findling JW, et al. The diagnosis of Cushing's syndrome: an endocrine society clinical practice guideline. J Clin Endocrinol Metab 2008; 93(5):1526–40.
18. Yanovski JA, Cutler GB Jr, Chrousos GP, et al. Corticotropin-releasing hormone stimulation following low-dose dexamethasone administration. A new test to distinguish Cushing's syndrome from pseudo-Cushing's states. JAMA 1993; 269(17):2232–8.
19. Batista DL, Courcoutsakis N, Riar J, et al. Severe obesity confounds the interpretation of low-dose dexamethasone test combined with the administration of ovine corticotrophin-releasing hormone in childhood Cushing syndrome. J Clin Endocrinol Metab 2008;93(11):4323–30.
20. Louiset E, Stratakis CA, Perraudin V, et al. The paradoxical increase in cortisol secretion induced by dexamethasone in primary pigmented nodular adrenocortical disease involves a glucocorticoid receptor-mediated effect of dexamethasone on protein kinase a catalytic subunits. J Clin Endocrinol Metab 2009; 94(7):2406–13.
21. Chrousos GP, Schulte HM, Oldfield EH, et al. The corticotropin-releasing factor stimulation test. An aid in the evaluation of patients with Cushing's syndrome. N Engl J Med 1984;310(10):622–6.
22. Batista D, Courkoutsakis NA, Oldfield EH, et al. Detection of adrenocorticotropin-secreting pituitary adenomas by magnetic resonance imaging in children and adolescents with Cushing disease. J Clin Endocrinol Metab 2005;90(9):5134–40.
23. Oldfield EH, Doppman JL, Nieman LK, et al. Petrosal sinus sampling with and without corticotropin-releasing hormone for the differential diagnosis of Cushing's syndrome. N Engl J Med 1991;325(13):897–905.
24. Batista D, Gennari M, Riar J, et al. An assessment of petrosal sinus sampling for localization of pituitary microadenomas in children with Cushing disease. J Clin Endocrinol Metab 2006;91(1):221–4.
25. Batista DL, Oldfield EH, Keil MF, et al. Postoperative testing to predict recurrent Cushing disease in children. J Clin Endocrinol Metab 2009;94(8):2757–65.
26. Powell AC, Stratakis CA, Patronas NJ, et al. Operative management of Cushing syndrome secondary to micronodular adrenal hyperplasia. Surgery 2008; 143(6):750–8.
27. Lodish M, Dunn SV, Sinaii N, et al. Recovery of the hypothalamic-pituitary-adrenal axis in children and adolescents after surgical cure of Cushing's disease. J Clin Endocrinol Metab 2012;97(5):1483–91.
28. Merke DP, Giedd JN, Keil MF, et al. Children experience cognitive decline despite reversal of brain atrophy one year after resolution of Cushing syndrome. J Clin Endocrinol Metab 2005;90(5):2531–6.
29. Keil MF, Merke DP, Gandhi R, et al. Quality of life in children and adolescents 1-year after cure of Cushing syndrome: a prospective study. Clin Endocrinol (Oxf) 2009;71(3):326–33.

Pubertal Disorders and Bone Maturation

Liora Lazar, MD[a,b], Moshe Phillip, MD[a,b],*

KEYWORDS

- Bone age • Skeletal maturation • Pubertal growth spurt • Normal puberty
- Precocious puberty • Delayed puberty

KEY POINTS

- In normal puberty, the lack of correlation between bone age (BA) and the timing of pubertal events and the accelerated bone maturation rate associated with the rapid phase of growth should be recognized as normal, and should not be attributed to any pathology.
- In precocious puberty (PP), the degree of BA advancement at diagnosis cannot always serve as an accurate marker of the pubertal stage, especially in boys. Serial BA assessments may differentiate between patients with rapidly progressing and nonsustained PP.
- In PP, BA is helpful in reaching decisions regarding treatment. The finding of accelerated bone maturation rate and deterioration in adult height prediction (AHP) with time reassures the physician that treatment is indeed necessary. Repeated BA assessments and AHP facilitate evaluation of the efficacy of the treatment modalities throughout the treatment period and following its cessation.
- In delayed puberty, BA is helpful in distinguishing between functional and permanent hypogonadism, in the interpretation of the hormonal evaluation, and in monitoring the effect of therapeutic interventions.
- AHP has been validated only in healthy and normally growing children, and height predictions may be less accurate in children with atypical puberty. In normal puberty AHP is relatively accurate. In precocious or delayed puberty, the precision of height prediction has proved to be unsatisfactory. It is generally overestimated in both untreated and treated children with either precocious or delayed puberty.
- Although BA assessment is a qualitative and not a quantitative measure, it serves to round out the clinical picture, providing important information that can aid the clinician in reaching a diagnosis, making treatment decisions, and monitoring treatment results.

Disclosure information: All authors have nothing to declare.
[a] The Jesse Z and Sara Lea Shafer Institute for Endocrinology and Diabetes, National Center for Childhood Diabetes, Schneider Children's Medical Center of Israel, 14 Kaplan Street, Petach Tikva 49202, Israel; [b] Sackler Faculty of Medicine, Tel Aviv University, Tel Aviv 69978, Israel
* Corresponding author.
E-mail address: mosheph@post.tau.ac.il

Endocrinol Metab Clin N Am 41 (2012) 805–825
http://dx.doi.org/10.1016/j.ecl.2012.08.003
0889-8529/12/$ – see front matter © 2012 Elsevier Inc. All rights reserved.

INTRODUCTION

Puberty is a complex process involving the activation and maturation of the hypothalamic-pituitary-gonadal (HPG) axis. The pubertal period is characterized by rapid changes in body size and shape that are sexually dimorphic. It begins with the appearance of secondary sexual characteristics and acceleration of growth, and ends with the acquisition of reproductive capability and the attainment of adult body habitus and final height.[1]

Clinical assessment of pubertal maturation status is based on Tanner's 5 developmental stages of breasts and pubic hair in girls and of pubic hair and genitalia in boys.[1–3] Pubertal growth spurt, representing 15% to 20% of adult height, is also a central feature among the remarkable physical changes occurring during puberty. As puberty approaches, growth velocity slows to a nadir before its acceleration during mid puberty. In girls, the timing of pubertal growth spurt is typically at early to mid puberty, the total height gain is about 25 cm, and the average peak height velocity (PHV), occurring at the age of 12 years, is 9 cm/y. Boys, on average, attain a PHV of 10.3 cm/y 2 years later than girls, at mid to late puberty, and gain approximately 28 cm in height through puberty. By the end of puberty, growth rate decelerates and soon after virtually ceases because of epiphyseal fusion.[1,4]

It has been well established that normal puberty follows a well-orchestrated pattern and has a predictable sequence. Yet age at onset of puberty differs in healthy children: the average age in girls is 9.5 to 10 years and in boys 11.5 to 12 years, but it may range from 8 to 13 years in girls and from 9 to 14 years in boys. Pubertal course, the rate of pubertal progression, and the timing and magnitude of PHV vary considerably as well.[1,5,6] Therefore, as chronologic age does not reflect the pubertal maturity status, pubertal onset and milestones should be related to the "biological" rather than the "chronologic" age.

Skeletal maturation may serve as an indicator of the biological age. Bone maturation is regulated by complex hormonal interactions involving the somatotropic, thyroid, adrenal, and gonadal axes. Throughout infancy, childhood, and puberty, the bones change in size and shape. As a child grows, the carpal and tarsal bones of the hands and feet and their epiphyses become calcified and appear on the radiographs. During puberty, bone maturation accelerates and the cartilaginous portions of the epiphyses become completely obliterated, demonstrating epiphyseal fusion.[7] This fusion is considered as occurring at bone age (BA) 15 in girls and 17 in boys. These changes in the growth plate often appear to parallel pubertal development. Conditions associated with delayed skeletal maturation also tend to delay the onset of puberty, whereas conditions that accelerate skeletal maturation tend to hasten the onset of puberty. Among the most common causes for markedly accelerated bone maturation are prolonged exposure to elevated levels of estradiol, testosterone, or adrenal androgens, as in PP,[8] congenital adrenal hyperplasia[9,10] or persistent hyperthyroidism.[11] Mildly advanced BA is found in precocious adrenarche[12] and to a lesser extent in premature thelarche,[13] whilst less prominent advancement is associated with overweight from a young age,[14] constitutional tall stature,[15] and various bone dysplasias.[16] Conversely, conditions that delay skeletal maturation, such as chronic disease and malnutrition,[17,18] hypothyroidism,[19] constitutional delay,[20] and growth hormone (GH) deficiency,[21] delay the onset of puberty. Thus BA may play a pivotal role in the clinical evaluation and management of children with growth and/or pubertal disorders. However, clinicians must keep in mind the limitations of BA in view of several crucial questions regarding diagnosis and treatment of these conditions, to be addressed later.

A recent mini-review examined the role of skeletal maturity assessment in children with short and tall stature and with various endocrine disorders.[22] This review focuses on the association between bone maturation and pubertal development, and emphasizes the role of skeletal maturation in the evaluation of normal puberty and various pubertal disorders. Three topics are discussed:

1. The contribution of BA in evaluating children with normal, precocious and delayed puberty, and in distinguishing between normal pubertal variants and pubertal disorders
2. The value of BA in predicting adult height in normal puberty and in pubertal disorders
3. The role of BA in deciding whether to treat children with inadequate pubertal growth, and in monitoring the effect of various treatments on skeletal maturation during and following cessation of treatment

SKELETAL MATURATION
Bone Age Assessment

Skeletal age, or BA, is considered to be a surrogate marker of physiologic maturity. Determination of BA is based on assessment of the successive changes in the appearance and shape of the bones of the hand and wrist taking place from birth to maturity, as viewed in hand-wrist radiographs. Four parameters are examined: the width of the epiphysis, the appearance of ossification centers, the capping of the epiphysis, and the fusion of the epiphysis (**Fig. 1**). The hand-wrist radiograph is universally used for this purpose because the site is easily radiographed, with minimal gonadal and bone marrow exposure to the small dose of radiation, and permits evaluation of multiple cuboid and long bones in a single radiographic view.

In clinical practice, BA assessment is made by matching of the examined radiograph of the left hand and wrist with a reference set of standard hand images of healthy and normally growing children belonging to a comparable population. Because girls are physiologically more mature than boys at any given chronologic age, separate standards exist for girls and boys.[23] A single determination of BA informs the clinician about the relationship between chronologic age and skeletal maturation at a particular time. Successive BA evaluations indicate the child's skeletal

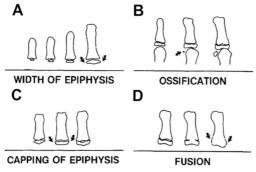

Fig. 1. Radiographic identification of skeletal maturity indicators. (*A*) Epiphysis equal in width to diaphysis. (*B*) Appearance of adductor sesamoid of the thumb. (*C*) Capping of epiphysis. (*D*) Fusion of epiphysis. (*Reprinted from* Fishman LS. Radiographic evaluation of skeletal maturation. A clinically oriented method based on hand-wrist films. Angle Orthod 1982;52(2):88–112; with permission.)

maturation rate. In healthy subjects BA should fall within 2 standard deviations (SDs) of reference norms.[1] A discrepancy between these 2 values indicates abnormalities in skeletal maturation.

The 2 most widely used methods for BA determination are (1) the Greulich and Pyle Atlas method[23] (derived from white children of upper socioeconomic class in 1931–1942) and (2) the Tanner-Whitehouse bone-scoring method (TW2)[24–26] (based on a sample of urban and rural children taken in the 1950s). When using the Greulich-Pyle method, the radiograph to be assessed is compared with the series of standard plates, and the age given to the standard plate that fits most closely is assigned as the BA of the child. The simplicity and speed with which a skeletal age can be assigned has made this method the most commonly used standard of reference for skeletal maturation worldwide. With the TW2 method each bone of the hand and wrist is matched with a set of 8 standard ages and its stage is rated, with the sum of the scores for all the bones representing the overall estimated BA. Scoring bone by bone makes the TW2 method potentially more accurate than the Greulich-Pyle atlas method, but it is consistently time consuming and may actually lead to a higher risk of error than that of Greulich-Pyle. It should be kept in mind that these 2 methods are very different and it is therefore necessary to use the same method in the follow-up of an individual, or in comparing different groups of patients. Each of these methods has its own drawbacks. Because the progression of BA with age, sex, and pubertal maturation differs in various populations the applicability of these standards to children of diverse ethnicity may be problematic. Also to be taken into consideration is that because these methods are based on manual BA determination, the assessment is necessarily subjective. Recently an automated system of BA measurement using computerized image analysis based on both Greulich-Pyle and TW2 has been cleared for clinical use in Europe. The use of this automated system was validated in healthy children and in children with various endocrine disorders. However, it has several limitations: BA range is restricted to 2 to 15 years for girls and 2.5 to 17 years for boys; it determines only 13 bones; it does not take into account the carpal bones; and the morphologic changes of the bones that may indicate bone disease or dysplasia are not recognized.[27]

Adult Height Prediction

BA is inversely associated with the remaining linear growth potential and is considered to be a functional marker of the decline in growth potential of the epiphyseal growth plate (EGP). This association is the basis for most height-prediction methods. For adult height prediction (AHP), 2 variables are needed: the child's current height and his BA. Over the years various methods for predicting adult height have been developed. Three methods are now in common use for AHP: those of Bayley and Pinneau (BP),[28] Roche, Wainer, and Thissen (RWT),[29] and Tanner and colleagues (TW).[24–26] The most recommended method is that of BP, which compares the hand-wrist radiograph with the BA atlas of Greulich and Pyle, each BA corresponding to a "percentage of adult height" found in a table included as an appendix in the Greulich-Pyle atlas. Separate tables are used for boys and girls because of the sex difference in timing of puberty. Slightly different percentages are used for children with unusually advanced or delayed bone maturation, as demonstrated in the "advanced" and "retarded" tables. To predict adult height, the present height of the examined child is divided by the "percent adult height." It should be kept in mind that AHP has been validated only in healthy and normally growing children, and height predictions may be less accurate in children with atypical growth, abnormal pubertal tempo, endocrine disorders, or bone abnormalities. In an attempt to improve the reliability of AHP, a new method based on automatic BA determination was recently developed.[30]

Epiphyseal Growth Plate Maturation and Fusion During Puberty

The osseous changes seen in the hand and wrist radiographs through the growth period are considered a reflection of ossification of the EGP. The EGP is a thin layer of cartilage entrapped between the epiphyseal and metaphyseal bone, at the distal ends of the long bones. The growth plate consists of 3 principal layers: resting zone, proliferative zone, and hypertrophic zone (**Fig. 2**). Longitudinal bone growth and maturation take place in the EGP through the process of endochondral bone formation, in which cartilage is first formed and then remodeled into bone tissue. This process entails the recruitment of chondrocytes in the resting zone of the growth plate cartilage to start active proliferation, followed by differentiation, apoptosis, and eventually mineralization and bone formation. The net effect is that new bone tissue is progressively created at the bottom of the growth plate, resulting in bone elongation.

Bone elongation and maturation during puberty are influenced by various hormones acting directly or indirectly on the EGP through several local growth factors, and by mechanisms intrinsic to the growth plate (**Fig. 3**).[31] The pubertal growth spurt results mainly from the synergistic effect of gonadal sex steroids, GH, and insulin-like growth factor I (IGF-I), all of which show a significant increase in serum levels during this period.[1] The increase in GH secretion is modulated by estrogens in both boys and girls,[31] whereas androgens influence the GH/IGF-I axis only after aromatization into estrogens.[32] Increased GH secretion augments circulating levels of IGF-I, inducing

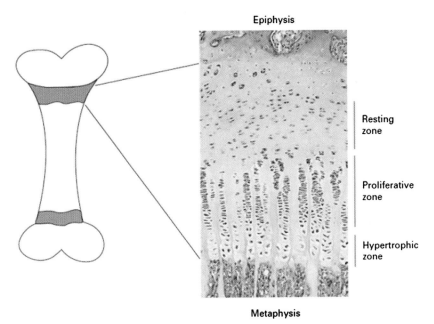

Fig. 2. Histology of the growth plate. The growth plate is a thin cartilage structure situated in the ends of tubular bones. It is commonly subdivided into 3 distinct zones: the resting, proliferative, and hypertrophic zones. (*Reprinted from* Nilsson O, Marino R, De Luca F, et al. Endocrine regulation of the growth plate. Horm Res 2005;64(4):157–65; with permission.)

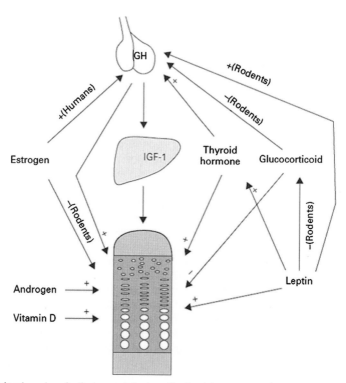

Fig. 3. Endocrine signals that regulate longitudinal bone growth. Arrows indicate direct action on the growth plate and indirect action by modulating other endocrine signals. +, stimulatory effect; −, inhibitory effect; GH, growth hormone; IGF, insulin-like growth factor. (*Reprinted from* Nilsson O, Marino R, De Luca F, et al. Endocrine regulation of the growth plate. Horm Res 2005;64(4):157–65; with permission.)

proliferation and differentiation of the chondrocytes in the EGP.[33] The serum GH levels may also have a direct stimulatory effect on the growth plate, mediated at least partially through local activation of the IGF system.[34]

Both androgens and estrogens appear to have a direct growth-modulating effect on the EGP by stimulating local production of IGF-I and other growth factors. Previous studies have demonstrated a dose-dependent stimulatory effect of estrogens in the EGP. Low estrogen concentrations, as detected at onset of puberty, stimulate chondrocyte growth in the proliferation zone, whereas high concentrations, found when puberty advances, induce apoptosis of hypertrophic chondrocytes, stimulate invasion of the growth plate by osteoblasts, and eventually lead to epiphyseal fusion and cessation of longitudinal growth.[35] Testosterone exerts its effect on the EPG through enhancement of the abundance and responsiveness of the IGF-I receptors in the growth plate chondrocytes rather than by a direct effect on their proliferation and differentiation. At least part of this effect is mediated by local stimulation of the IGF-I and IGF-I-receptor gene expression.[36]

Another important element of pubertal growth relates to the amount of body fat. Leptin, considered the link between adipose tissue and growth, plays a crucial role in pubertal growth, either by activating the leptin receptors in the growth plate or by stimulating IGF-I-receptor gene expression and abundance in the growth center, independent of the presence of GH.[37]

Regarding growth plate maturation and fusion, it is well established that estrogens are essential for epiphyseal closure in both males and females. This finding was confirmed with the recognition of 2 genetic disorders, estrogen deficiency due to mutations in the aromatase gene[38] and estrogen resistance due to mutations in the estrogen receptor-α (ERα) gene,[39] in both of which the growth plate fails to fuse, with persistence of growth into adulthood. By contrast, in the complete androgen insensitivity syndrome, in which only the estrogen receptor is functioning, affected XY females showed a normal pubertal growth spurt and epiphyseal fusion.[40] The estrogen effect in the growth plate is mediated by 2 estrogen receptors, ERα and ERβ, which are colocalized in the late-proliferating and early-hypertrophic zones. ERα is the dominant receptor; ERβ, which is able to heterodimerize with ERα, may have a role in fine-tuning the activity of ERα and acts as its negative regulator.[41] It could thus be speculated that the enhanced ERα-mediated signaling in the growth plate, leading to the EGP maturation and fusion, stems from the decreased activity of ERβ during late puberty. Recently a third estrogen receptor, GPR30, was identified as being expressed in the growth plate of both girls and boys, with expression localized to the resting and hypertrophic zones and absent from the proliferative zone. Its expression declines as puberty progresses.[42] These findings indicate that this receptor may also be involved in the modulation of pubertal growth.

The changes in the EGP observed through puberty are not attributed solely to the aforementioned hormonal changes. New evidence suggests that these may be due to a local mechanism within the growth plate. The EGP undergoes programmed senescence with age, as evidenced by reduced height of the growth plate and the decline in the chondrocyte proliferation rate occurring because of the gradual exhaustion of the finite proliferative capacity of stem-like cells in the resting zone of the EGP.[35]

It has been demonstrated that premature exposure of the EGP to high levels of estrogens, as present in precocious puberty (PP), accelerates its senescence and diminishes its elongation potential.[43]

Understanding the maturation processes within the EGP during puberty may contribute to a better assessment and a more accurate interpretation of BA readings during normal puberty and in pubertal disorders.

SKELETAL MATURATION IN NORMAL PUBERTY
The Role of BA Assessment in Normal Puberty

BA assessment in normal puberty should be used with caution. To begin with, an accurate BA assessment requires the use of the appropriate skeletal age standards for the given population. Previous studies have shown that in black and Hispanic adolescent girls and Asian and Hispanic adolescent boys, BA exceeds chronologic age by 9 to 11 months.[44,45] Hence, the most widely used standards are not applicable in these populations.

Recognition of the normal speed-up in skeletal age associated with the rapid phase of growth in puberty is also required. It is usually to be expected that in a healthy, normal child skeletal maturation will advance in parallel with chronologic age and with pubertal milestones, and that any deviation from this pattern may suggest an underlying clinical problem. This assumption, however, is incorrect for the years of puberty. Up to 2 years before the age of PHV, and for a short time thereafter, skeletal age advances more quickly than chronologic age.[44]

Physicians should also be aware that there is only a weak correlation between skeletal maturation and the timing of pubertal events. As already noted, although within the normal population most adolescents follow a predictable path through puberty, there is wide variation in age at onset of puberty and in timing, sequence, and tempo of pubertal maturation. This variability is not always reflected by the skeletal maturation rate. As early as 1974, Marshall[46] reported on variability in BA at onset of puberty in normal boys and girls, emphasizing that the correlation between onset of puberty with BA was no stronger than with chronologic age. In a more recent study, Flor-Cisneros and colleagues[47] found no correlation between the degree of skeletal advancement and the degree of pubertal progression in boys with normal onset of puberty.

It must be stressed that slightly delayed or advanced BA may be found in children undergoing a normal pubertal onset and course. Advanced skeletal maturation is prevalent among overweight adolescents[48] and patients with constitutional tall stature. Furthermore, it may also be present in children with no underlying medical problem or any endocrinopathy, and therefore would be considered idiopathic. In such cases, the growth pattern and pubertal development are usually normal and adult height is not compromised.[49] Hence during normal puberty, BA variations must be recognized as normal and should not be attributed to any pathologic aspects.

Adult Height Prediction in Normal Puberty

The equations used nowadays for predicting the adult height of a child, based on large numbers of normal children and, more importantly, on a sample that also includes relatively large numbers of very tall, very short, and very growth-delayed children,[24–26,28] have improved the reliability of height prediction in normal children. Height prediction in most children older than 8 years in girls and 11 years in boys is relatively accurate. For boys at onset of puberty, 95% of the predictions lie within ± 8 cm of the real value, falling to ± 6 cm at age 15 years. For premenarcheal girls the predictions lie within about ± 6 cm at age 8 years and reach ± 4 cm at 13 years. For postmenarcheal girls the predictions are substantially more consistent.[25] At onset of puberty, AHP in tall children is more precise in girls than in boys, and for both sexes the prediction becomes increasingly accurate with advancing age.[50]

The Role of BA in Management of Extremely Short and Tall Children

The definition of extremes of growth is based on the normal variance of growth within the reference population. In general, a child whose height differs by more than 2 SDs from the population mean is considered either too tall or too short. Very short and very tall adolescents tend to seek medical help to evaluate height prognosis and ultimately try to "normalize" adult height if they see the estimate as unfavorable. By providing information on skeletal maturation, BA assessment is commonly used in deciding whether to treat these children, and in monitoring the effect of the various treatments on skeletal maturation rate.

Children with extremely short height prognosis

In adolescents with normal puberty but poor height prognosis (idiopathic short stature [ISS] or persistent short stature after intrauterine growth retardation [IUGR]), it was assumed that by inhibiting estrogen biosynthesis the skeletal maturation rate would decline, the "prepubertal" growth phase would be extended, and consequently the final height (FHt) would be improved. This assumption led to the use of gonadotropin-releasing hormone analogues (GnRHa) for suppression of puberty, and/or of aromatase inhibitors for inhibiting the conversion of androgens to estrogens. The efficacy of the treatment modalities was evaluated by repeated BA assessments and AHP throughout the treatment period. There are only a few studies[51,52] presenting FHt data in children with ISS and normal puberty treated by GnRHa, and most of these reported only a modest improvement of predicted or attained adult height following lengthy treatment. Furthermore, these studies found that ISS was associated with adverse psychosocial consequences related to pubertal delay as well as decreased accretion of bone mineral content. The introduction of treatment with a combination of GH and GnRHa showed a better pubertal growth but only a relatively small improvement in FHt.[53–55] Therefore, combined GH and GnRHa treatment is considered only in individual patients with extremely poor AHP.[55]

Aromatase inhibitors (letrozole or anastrozole) are increasingly used to promote growth in peripubertal and pubertal boys with growth disorders. Results from several studies showed that aromatase inhibitors effectively slowed BA advancement and increased AHP without stopping the pubertal development and attenuating the pubertal growth spurt.[56] However, because of the lack of substantial safety data regarding aromatase inhibitor treatment in children and adolescents, including the effects of treatment on skeletal health and vertebral body morphology,[57] their use outside a research setting is currently not recommended.

Children with extremely tall height prognosis

Constitutional tall stature, a variant of the normal pattern of childhood growth and development, is defined as a condition whereby the height of an individual is 2 SDs above the corresponding mean height for a normal subject of the same age and sex, in the absence of pathologic causes of tall stature. Medical treatment of children and adolescents with constitutional tall stature is controversial. Treatment was common in the past, particularly for girls, but is now strongly discouraged except in extreme cases in view of increased cultural acceptance of tall stature, the unsatisfactory outcome, and the recognition of side effects of treatment.[50,58]

High doses of sex steroids (estrogen in girls and testosterone in boys) have been used in the treatment of tall children in an attempt to promote premature epiphyseal fusion and reduce the adult height.[58] In girls estrogen treatment is usually started when BA ranges between 10 and 12 years, and is not indicated with BA of 14 to 15 years.[50] In boys treatment is more effective when started when the BA is less than 14 to 15 years of age. It should be kept in mind that initiation of treatment in a more advanced BA can accelerate growth rate.[50] In both girls and boys, BA assessment is also mandatory before discontinuation of treatment. Treatment should be continued until the epiphyses have fused because posttreatment growth may be substantial if cessation is premature.

SKELETAL MATURATION IN PRECOCIOUS PUBERTY

PP is defined as the onset of secondary sexual development before the age of 8 years in girls and 9 years in boys.[1] PP is a heterogeneous condition with regard to its underlying etiology and course. It has been classified into 3 categories: (1) gonadotropin-dependent or central precocious puberty (CPP), caused in more than 80% of the patients by an idiopathic activation of the gonadotropic axis—in the remainder, central nervous system (CNS) anomalies or tumors have been found to be the underlying cause; (2) gonadotropin-independent or peripheral precocious puberty, caused by peripheral secretion of sex hormones from either the gonads or adrenal glands, by ectopic human chorionic gonadotropin production by a germ cell tumor, or by exogenous sources of sex steroids; and (3) incomplete precocious puberty, consisting of isolated breast development (premature thelarche) or isolated pubic or axillary hair development mediated by androgens produced in the adrenal glands (precocious adrenarche).[1] The course of puberty also varies, its spectrum comprising nonsustained, slowly progressive, and rapidly progressive forms. Nonsustained or slowly progressive PP is characterized by either stabilization of pubertal signs or slow progression; the pubertal growth potential is preserved and the adult height is not affected. Rapidly progressing PP is characterized by rapid development of the secondary sexual characteristics, early menarche in girls, accelerated growth velocity and tall stature at diagnosis but ultimately compromised adult stature, and adverse psychosocial outcomes. These adverse effects may be prevented by appropriate treatment aimed at halting the advancement of secondary sexual characteristics and slowing the EGP maturation rate so as to achieve a normal FHt.[1]

The major concern at initial evaluation is to identify the underlying etiology and to exclude CNS or gonadal neoplasms. The secondary concern is to define the pace of pubertal progression and thereby to select the patients who should be treated.

The Role of BA Assessment in Diagnosis of CPP

In CPP, the premature exposure of the EGP to sex hormones accelerates the bone maturation rate so that BA of patients with CPP is generally more advanced than their chronologic age.[1] BA assessment at diagnosis may differentiate between patients with rapidly progressing CPP and other pubertal variants. Rapidly progressing CPP is characterized by rapid bone maturation rate, whereas in nonsustained or slowly progressive CPP it is only slightly accelerated. Thus BA advancement in rapidly progressing CPP is greater than 2 SD, whereas in nonsustained CPP it is only 1 to 2 SD above chronologic age.[59–62] The degree of BA advancement cannot always serve as an accurate marker of the pubertal pace. BA may be only slightly advanced when the diagnosis is made close to the onset of puberty. Moreover, in boys, accelerated bone maturation normally occurs in advanced pubertal stages (Tanner 4–5); when diagnosed at early stages of puberty, the BA may still correspond to the chronologic age.[62]

Prediction of FHt is an important tool in the initial workup of CPP. The observation that AHP is compromised compared with target height obliges medical intervention. In historical untreated CPP patients, the precision of height prediction using either the "accelerated tables" or the "average tables" was unsatisfactory.[63,64] A systematic overestimation of FHt between 3.7 and 5.9 cm was recorded in girls,[63,65] while in the relatively few data available for boys it was even greater.[62] This inaccuracy may stem from the fact that the most widely used methods, the Bayley-Pinneau and TW, were based on children with no underlying endocrinopathies.

The Role of BA Assessment at Initiation of GnRHa Treatment

The decision as to whether to treat CPP with a GnRHa agonist depends on the child's age, the rate of pubertal progression, height velocity, and the estimated adult height as determined from the rate of BA advancement. Most pediatric endocrinologists agree that precocious age at onset of puberty, fast pubertal development, accelerated growth rate, and BA advancement greater than 2 SDs warrant treatment. The pace of bone maturation should also be considered,[61–63,66] with the occasional requirement of repeated BA monitoring before initiation of treatment; the finding of accelerated bone maturation rate will reassure the physician that treatment is indeed necessary. The observation that predicted FHt is progressively deteriorating with time and that FHt might be compromised calls for medical intervention as well.

Age at onset of CPP is an important predictor of FHt outcome. A satisfactory FHt is achieved when age at onset of puberty is less than 5 to 6 years and when GnRHa treatment is initiated soon thereafter.[67] The effect of treatment on FHt in girls with onset of puberty at ages 6 to 8 years is controversial,[68–74] and in girls with pubertal onset between 8 and 9 years no benefit is achieved.[75–77] These findings may be attributed to the fact that accelerated senescence of the EGP caused by exposure to estrogens will decrease the elongation potential of the bones.[35]

In boys, assessment of the BA must take into consideration that acceleration of the bone maturation rate occurs in the later pubertal stages. Hence, the decision to institute suppressive therapy should be based on the rate of pubertal progression, that is, the increase in testicular volume and advancement of secondary sexual characteristics associated with the increase in testosterone levels, rather than on growth rate and BA advancement.[62]

The Role of BA in Assessing Efficacy of GnRHa Treatment

Slowing BA advancement and prolongation of the growth period are the primary goals for improving adult height in CPP. BA should therefore be assessed at periodic intervals (approximately every 6–12 months) to determine effectiveness of therapy in arresting skeletal maturation. On institution of treatment, bone maturation rate may at first accelerate because GnRHa initially act to stimulate gonadotropin secretion. A few weeks later, on pituitary desensitization, skeletal maturation is attenuated (0.5–1 years/y).[69] At an even later stage of treatment BA advancement may even freeze.[70–73] Rapid BA advancement during treatment requires prompt reassessment. In boys the response to GnRHa generally resembles that of girls with regard to attenuation of growth and bone maturation rates,[71] but during the first year of therapy there reportedly was a greater decline in BA advancement.[78]

FHt Prediction and the Role of BA Assessment at Cessation of GnRHa Treatment and Following Discontinuation of Treatment

The appropriate time for discontinuation of GnRHa treatment is also related to BA. All studies have shown that BA at the end of treatment correlated negatively with height gain after treatment (**Fig. 4**).[69,70] In 1999, Carel and colleagues[72] reported that an optimal residual growth capacity was achieved in girls when BA at cessation was 12 to 12.5 years. Based on these data, the policy of many endocrinology clinics is to interrupt treatment in girls with sexual precocity, whether diagnosed early (<6 years) or later (6–8 or 8–9 years), at the BA recommended above. However, the achieved FHt was generally less than the FHt prediction at discontinuation of treatment, particularly

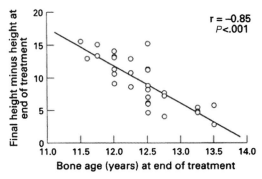

Fig. 4. Final height minus height at end of triptorelin treatment as a function of bone age (years) at the end of triptorelin treatment in girls (N = 31). (*Reprinted from* Oostdijk W, Rikken B, Schreuder S, et al. Final height in central precocious puberty after long term treatment with a slow release GnRH agonist. Arch Dis Child 1996;75(4):292–7; with permission of the BMJ Publishing Group Ltd.)

in girls with pubertal onset at older than 6 years. In 2007, the authors' group[74] showed that the reduced height gain was related to the accelerated bone maturation rate and earlier epiphyseal fusion of girls with sexual precocity diagnosed after the age of 6 years (**Fig. 5**). The difference in residual growth to FHt was related to the senescence of the EGP before initiation of treatment. Thus, because of the deceleration of the bone maturation rate, the improved height prediction throughout the treatment period proved to have been overly optimistic.

The criteria for discontinuation of treatment in boys have been the subject of debate. In normal boys, PHV occurs around the chronologic age of 13.5 years, which corresponds to early mid puberty in boys and is associated with a satisfactory posttreatment growth spurt. This BA is therefore recommended for GnRHa treatment interruption.[71] Improved FHt prediction during GnRHa treatment was noted in boys as well but, as in girls, their achieved FHt was significantly lower than the predicted FHt (**Fig. 6**).[70,74,78] Hence, the BP method is not reliable for FHt prediction, neither in boys nor in girls older than 6 years at onset of puberty, and the actual improvement in height prognosis in most treated children is less than expected.[72]

The Role of BA Assessment in Incomplete Precocious Puberty

Incomplete PP consists of premature thelarche and precocious adrenarche, both variants of normal puberty. BA is only slightly advanced in these 2 conditions. If the BA is normal or only marginally advanced and growth rate is not accelerated, an extensive evaluation is usually not required. Nonetheless, monitoring of children with these conditions is needed to ensure that they do not develop CPP.

Premature thelarche is characterized by isolated breast development, absence of other signs of puberty, normal growth rate, and normal or only slight BA advancement. Most cases are idiopathic and present around 2 years of age (but may start at birth), and either remit spontaneously or progress very slowly. Premature thelarche may progress to true isosexual PP, present in 14% to 20% of these children.[13,79] To identify these patients regular follow-up is required, with examination for signs pubertal development and determination of growth rate and BA. An accelerated height velocity or bone maturation rate would suggest progressive puberty.

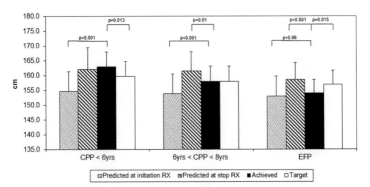

Fig. 5. Final height of 115 girls with sexual precocity treated by GnRHa predicted at initiation and at discontinuation of gonadotropin-suppressive therapy, versus achieved target height. CPP, central precocious puberty; EFP, early fast puberty; RX, therapy. (*Reprinted from* Lazar L, Padoa A, Phillip M. Growth pattern and final height after cessation of gonadotropin-suppressive therapy in girls with central sexual precocity. J Clin Endocrinol Metab 2007;92(9):3483–9; with permission of the Endocrine Society.)

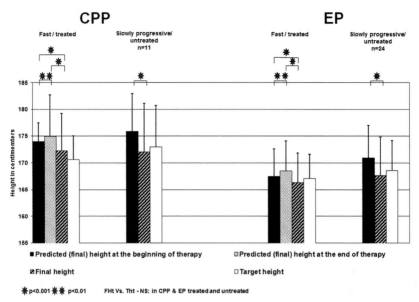

Fig. 6. Predicted and achieved final height versus target height in 66 boys with sexual precocity, treated (11 central precocious puberty [CPP], 20 early puberty [EP]) and untreated (11 CPP, 24 EP). (*Reprinted from* Lazar L, Pertzelan A, Weintrob N, et al. Sexual precocity in boys: accelerated versus slowly progressive puberty gonadotropin-suppressive therapy and final height. J Clin Endocrinol Metab 2001;86(9):4127–32; with permission of the Endocrine Society.)

Precocious adrenarche refers to the isolated appearance of pubic and/or axillary hair with no evidence of gonadarche before the age of 8 years in girls and 9 years in boys when androgen-producing tumors, steroidogenic enzyme defects, and central puberty have been excluded.[12] Bone elongation and maturation rates tend to be above average, as reflected by relatively tall stature and BA advancement. Girls with precocious adrenarche who were born AGA are characterized by a broad spectrum of clinical manifestations at presentation. However, the clinical outcome of these girls is regarded as benign, characterized by a slow progression of bone maturation rate, lack of virilization, normal onset and progression of sexual development, and uncompromised adult height irrespective of the extent of adrenarche at presentation. Adult height prediction is unreliable in this population.[80]

SKELETAL MATURATION IN DELAYED PUBERTY

Delayed puberty is defined as the absence of secondary sexual characteristics (testicular enlargement in boys or breast development in girls), at an age that is 2 to 2.5 SDs later than the population mean (traditionally, the age of 14 years in boys and 12–13 years in girls). Delayed puberty usually results from inadequate gonadal steroid secretion owing to a variety of hypothalamic, pituitary, and gonadal disorders.[1] It is generally categorized into 2 groups: (1) primary gonadal failure due to various gonadal diseases, characterized by low sex hormones and elevated gonadotropin levels; and (2) secondary hypogonadism owing to hypothalamic dysfunction, hypopituitarism, or hyperprolactinemia, characterized by low sex hormones and gonadotropin levels. Impaired secretion and/or action of hypothalamic gonadotropin-releasing hormone

(GnRH) is the most frequent underlying cause of secondary hypogonadism. It can be functional, as in constitutional delay of growth and puberty (CDGP), chronic illness, excessive exercise, malnutrition, stress, and due to medications, or related to associated pathology, as with hypothalamic and pituitary tumors (especially craniopharyngioma), genetic causes (hypogonadotropic hypogonadism without or with anosmia [Kallmann syndrome]), and idiopathic isolated hypogonadotropic hypogonadism (HH).[1]

Diagnosis of CDGP is essentially a diagnosis of exclusion, when no underlying conditions can define the delay and sexual maturation occurs spontaneously before the age of 18 years. Patients with CDGP are healthy overall, with delayed onset of puberty but normal progression, a slightly reduced pubertal growth spurt, but uncompromised FHt when compared with the target height. There is generally a history of delayed growth and development throughout childhood, including short stature, but a relatively normal growth rate.[1,20,81]

In children with primary gonadal failure or permanent hypogonadism, bone elongation and maturation proceed uninhibited through childhood. During puberty, growth acceleration and epiphyseal fusion fail to occur, and disproportionately long extremities (eunuchoid habitus) may develop.[1,81] The syndrome of gonadal dysgenesis (GD) is an exception to this growth pattern. In GD the stunted growth already observed in early childhood is not attributed to the primary gonadal failure but to skeletal defects stemming from the lack of a second *SHOX* gene on the X chromosome.[82] In patients with CDGP or functional HH caused by underlying disease, growth retardation and delayed BA already become manifest before the expected age of pubertal onset. Because most of these disorders have in common a functional defect in GnRH secretion and/or its action, no single test reliably distinguishes patients with CDGP (who will eventually progress spontaneously through puberty) from patients with other causes of delayed puberty, particularly isolated HH. The most valuable components of an assessment are a focused history and physical examination, and observation over time.[1,81]

The Role of BA Assessment in Evaluation of Children with Delayed Puberty

BA radiographs are frequently helpful and should be routinely performed in children with growth and/or puberty retardation, because onset of puberty normally corresponds with a BA range of 11 to 12.5 years in boys and 9.5 to 10 years in girls.[1] Although the degree of BA delay per se is not diagnostic, determination of BA at the initial evaluation may permit differentiation between CDGP and isolated HH. A BA delay of more than 2 "years" has arbitrarily been used as an inclusion criterion for CDGP.[83,84] BA of patients with CDGP is generally appropriate to their reduced stature and to their stage of pubertal development. Their BA rarely progresses beyond 12 to 13.5 years without the presence of pubertal levels of gonadal steroids. By contrast, in patients with isolated HH, BA is usually slightly delayed and normal pubertal BA (older than or equal to 12 to 13 years) can be attained without evidence of puberty.[81] Assessment of the patient's growth pattern and skeletal maturation rate up to the time of evaluation might also be helpful because in patients with CDGP, growth rate and BA are delayed from early childhood.[1,20,81] When delayed skeletal maturation is associated with a reduced growth rate, endocrine disorders, including GH deficiency, hypothyroidism, and chronic systemic diseases, must be considered. However, it should be noted that with these conditions it may take some time before delay of the bone maturation rate. A BA consistent with chronologic age does not rule out the possibility of a recent onset of underlying diseases. In an obese child, delayed BA and growth retardation may point to Cushing syndrome or disease.[85] Obese girls may display advanced BA and early puberty, whereas in obese boys BA may be relatively retarded and onset of puberty quite delayed.[86] In girls with GD, BA appears to be only slightly delayed until the age of about 10 years, after which the rate of skeletal maturation considerably decreases and the delay in BA becomes more pronounced, in accordance with the estrogen deficiency.[82]

The Role of BA Assessment in Interpretation of GnRH Stimulation Test in Delayed Puberty

Stimulated levels of luteinizing hormone and follicle-stimulating hormone in the pubertal range following GnRH administration indicate that the HPG axis has been reactivated and that secondary sexual development is likely to occur. In cases of central delayed puberty, prepubertal values following GnRH stimulation may be observed at initial evaluation in both CDGP and isolated HH. Hence, GnRH stimulation testing does not help to distinguish between the 2 conditions. However, BA assessment may contribute to the interpretation of the GnRH stimulation test. A BA of 11 years in girls and 13 years in boys may be considered the threshold to expect the pubertal gonadotropin response.[87] Hence a low gonadotropin response to GnRH stimulation in the presence of a BA above 11 years in girls and 13 years in boys may suggest the diagnosis of isolated HH.

The Role of BA Assessment at Initiation of Therapy

Most patients with CDGP attain FHt within their target height range without any medical intervention. Short-term hormonal therapy with testosterone in boys and with estrogen in girls may be appropriate when the pubertal delay is severe or the patient's psychosocial concerns about the delay play a prominent role that cannot be addressed by reassurance and education alone. The treatment of CDGP or hypogonadism aims to induce development of sex characteristics and acceleration of the growth rate, with optimization of adult stature and mitigation of psychosocial difficulties. In most such patients it is difficult to distinguish between isolated HH and CDGP, for which reason the initial therapeutic approach is similar for both disorders. Therapy is generally initiated in girls older than 12 years and in boys older than 14 years with a BA of more than 12.5 years.[88] Short-term hormonal therapy, with testosterone in boys (long-acting testosterone esters, 50–150 mg per month during 6 months)[88–90] and low doses of estrogen in girls,[91] does not appear to have any long-term sequelae except for the potential skeletal maturation that may result in some loss of adult height and which necessitates frequent monitoring of BA during therapy.

For a subset of patients with CDGP, short stature can be more worrisome than delayed puberty. Treatment with GH may improve adult height and does not induce epiphyseal closure, but its use remains questionable in patients with CDGP.[92] Aromatase inhibitors are another potential therapeutic approach, as they delay the EGP fusion,[93,94] but in view of the possible adverse effects this treatment must be considered with caution.[57,94]

Treatment of girls with GD consists of GH administered throughout the growth period and estrogen replacement therapy at late puberty. Estrogen replacement should not be initiated early, as it may lead to accelerated bone maturation rate and compromise the adult height.[82,95]

Height Prediction in Children with CDGP

AHP is an important part of counseling in CDGP, particularly when short stature is a component of the presentation. However, one should be aware that the BP tables overestimate adult height in patients with CDGP if BA is delayed by more than 2 years.[96]

SUMMARY

In the evaluation of pubertal development, the chronologic age often fails to provide a clear picture of the possible variations in maturation rate. BA, by reflecting the stage of EGP maturation, indicates more clearly than chronologic age how far an individual has progressed toward full maturity and serves as a predictor of the potential for further growth. Although BA assessment does not identify a specific diagnosis, single or serial skeletal age estimations help the clinician to confirm the diagnosis of normal puberty and normal pubertal variants such as CDGP, premature therlache, and precocious adrenarche. BA can aid in the clinical workup of children whose sexual maturation is early or delayed, in reaching decisions regarding treatment, and in monitoring the effect of various treatments on the skeletal maturation rate during treatment and following its cessation. Adult height prediction also relies on assessment of skeletal maturity. However, because all height-predicting methods are based on data obtained from normal children, its applicability in patients with delayed or PP, particularly during or following GnRHa treatment, is not always reliable.

Other important caveats concerning BA assessment include intraobserver variance and lack of skeletal age standards for the studied population. The precision of the procedure is expected to be enhanced by the future development of techniques for scanning radiographs combined with computer analysis.

Although BA is considered a qualitative rather than a quantitative measure, it serves to round out the clinical picture, providing information without which diagnosis could not be achieved. Its complementary role is invaluable in diagnosis, treatment decisions, and treatment monitoring, as long as its limitations are recognized.

ACKNOWLEDGMENTS

The authors thank Dr Yael Lebenthal and Dr Tal Oron for critical reading of the review.

REFERENCES

1. Grumbach MM, Styne DM. Puberty: ontogeny, neuroendocrinology, physiology and disorders. In: Melmed S, Polonsky KS, Larsen PR, et al, editors. Williams' textbook of endocrinology. 12th edition. Philadelphia: W.B. Saunders Co; 2011. p. 1055–201.
2. Marshall WA, Tanner JM. Variations in the pattern of pubertal changes in girls. Arch Dis Child 1969;44(235):291–303.
3. Marshall WA, Tanner JM. Variations in the pattern of pubertal changes in boys. Arch Dis Child 1970;45(239):13–23.
4. Tanner JM, Whitehouse RH, Marubini E, et al. The adolescent growth spurt of boys and girls of the Harpenden growth study. Ann Hum Biol 1976;3(2):109–26.
5. Palmert MR, Boepple PA. Variation in the timing of puberty: clinical spectrum and genetic investigation. J Clin Endocrinol Metab 2001;86(6):2364–8.
6. Parent AS, Teilmann G, Juul A, et al. The timing of normal puberty and the age limits of sexual precocity: variations around the world, secular trends, and changes after migration. Endocr Rev 2003;24(5):668–93.
7. Hochberg Z. Endocrine control of skeletal maturation. Basel (Switzerland): Karger; 2002.
8. Brauner R, Adan L, Malandry A, et al. Adult height in girls with idiopathic true precocious puberty. J Clin Endocrinol Metab 1994;79(2):415–20.

9. Speiser PW, White PC. Congenital adrenal hyperplasia. N Engl J Med 2003; 349(8):776–88.
10. New MI. Extensive clinical experience: nonclassical 21-hydroxylase deficiency. J Clin Endocrinol Metab 2006;91(11):4205–14.
11. Schlesinger S, MacGillivray MH, Munschauer RW. Acceleration of growth and bone maturation in childhood thyrotoxicosis. J Pediatr 1973;83(2):233–6.
12. Ibañez L, Virdis R, Potau N, et al. Natural history of premature pubarche: an auxological study. J Clin Endocrinol Metab 1992;74(2):254–7.
13. Volta C, Bernasconi S, Cisternino M, et al. Isolated premature thelarche and thelarche variant: clinical and auxological follow-up of 119 girls. J Endocrinol Invest 1998;21(3):180–3.
14. Russell DL, Keil MF, Bonat SH, et al. The relation between skeletal maturation and adiposity in African American and Caucasian children. J Pediatr 2001;139(6): 844–8.
15. Dickerman Z, Loewinger J, Laron Z. The pattern of growth in children with constitutional tall stature from birth to age 9 years. A longitudinal study. Acta Paediatr Scand 1984;73(4):530–6.
16. Clark RN. Congenital dysplasias and dwarfism. Pediatr Rev 1990;12(5):149–59.
17. Kulin HE, Bwibo N, Mutie D, et al. The effect of chronic childhood malnutrition on pubertal growth and development. Am J Clin Nutr 1982;36(3):527–36.
18. Alvear J, Artaza C, Vial M, et al. Physical growth and bone age of survivors of protein energy malnutrition. Arch Dis Child 1986;61(3):257–62.
19. Pantsiouou S, Stanhope R, Uruena M, et al. Growth prognosis and growth after menarche in primary hypothyroidism. Arch Dis Child 1991;66(7):838–40.
20. Sedlmeyer IL, Palmert MR. Delayed puberty: analysis of a large case series from an academic center. J Clin Endocrinol Metab 2002;87(4):1613–20.
21. Tanner JM, Whitehouse RH. A note on the bone age at which patients with true isolated growth hormone deficiency enter puberty. J Clin Endocrinol Metab 1975;41(4):788–90.
22. Martin DD, Wit JM, Hochberg Z, et al. The use of bone age in clinical practice— part 1 & part 2. Horm Res Paediatr 2011;76(1):1–16.
23. Greulich W, Pyle S. Radiographic atlas of the skeletal development of the hand and wrist. 2nd edition. Stanford (CA): Stanford University Press; 1959.
24. Tanner JM, Whitehouse RH, Marshall WA, et al. Assessment of skeletal maturity and prediction of adult height (TW2 method). London: Academic Press; 1975.
25. Tanner JM, Landt KW, Cameron N, et al. Prediction of adult height from height and bone age in childhood. A new system of equations (TW Mark II) based on a sample including very tall and very short children. Arch Dis Child 1983; 58(10):767–76.
26. Tanner JM, Healy M, Goldstein H, et al. Assessment of skeletal maturity and prediction of adult height (TW3 method). 3rd edition. London: WB Saunders; 2001.
27. Thodberg HH. Clinical review: an automated method for determination of bone age. J Clin Endocrinol Metab 2009;94(7):2239–44.
28. Bayley N, Pinneau SR. Tables for predicting adult height from skeletal age: revised for use with the Greulich-Pyle hand standards. J Pediatr 1952;40(4): 423–41.
29. Roche AF, Wainer H, Thissen D. The RWT method for the prediction of adult stature. Pediatrics 1975;56(6):1027–33.
30. Thodberg HH, Neuhof J, Ranke MB, et al. Validation of bone age methods by their ability to predict adult height. Horm Res Paediatr 2010;74(1):15–22.

31. Nilsson O, Marino R, De Luca F, et al. Endocrine regulation of the growth plate. Horm Res 2005;64(4):157–65.
32. Veldhuis JD, Metzger DL, Martha PM Jr, et al. Estrogen and testosterone, but not a nonaromatizable androgen, direct network integration of hypothalamo-somatotrope (Growth Hormone)-insulin-like growth factor I axis in the human: evidence from pubertal pathophysiology and sex-steroid replacement. J Clin Endocrinol Metab 1997;82(10):3414–20.
33. Luna A, Wilson D, Wibbelsman C, et al. Somatomedins in adolescence; a cross sectional study of the effect of puberty on plasma insulin-like growth factor I and II levels. J Clin Endocrinol Metab 1983;57(2):268–71.
34. Isaksson OG, Lindahl A, Nilsson A, et al. Mechanism of the stimulatory effect of growth hormone on longitudinal bone growth. Endocr Rev 1987;8(4):426–38.
35. Weise M, De-Levi S, Barnes KM, et al. Effects of estrogen on growth plate senescence and epiphyseal fusion. Proc Natl Acad Sci U S A 2001;98(12):6871–6.
36. Phillip M, Maor G, Assa S, et al. Testosterone stimulates growth of tibial epiphyseal growth plate and insulin-like growth factor-I-receptor abundance and growth in hypophysectomized and castrated rats. Endocrine 2001;16(1):1–6.
37. Maor G, Rochberger M, Segev Y, et al. Leptin acts as a growth factor on the chondrocytes of skeletal growth center. J Bone Miner Res 2002;17(6):1034–43.
38. Morishima A, Grumbach MM, Simpson ER, et al. Aromatase deficiency in male and female siblings caused by a novel mutation and the physiological role of estrogens. J Clin Endocrinol Metab 1995;80(12):3689–98.
39. Smith EP, Boyd J, Frank GR, et al. Estrogen resistance caused by a mutation in the estrogen-receptor gene in a man. N Engl J Med 1994;331(16):1056–61.
40. Zachmann M, Prader A, Sobel EH, et al. Indirect evidence for the importance of estrogens in pubertal growth of girls. J Pediatr 1986;108(5 Pt 1):694–7.
41. Nilsson LO, Boman A, Sävendahl L, et al. Demonstration of estrogen receptor-β immunoreactivity in human growth plate cartilage. J Clin Endocrinol Metab 1999;84(1):370–3.
42. Chagin AS, Sävendahl L. GPR30 estrogen receptor expression in the growth plate declines as puberty progresses. J Clin Endocrinol Metab 2007;92(12):4873–7.
43. Weise M, Flor A, Barnes KM, et al. Determinants of growth during gonadotropin-releasing hormone analog therapy for precocious puberty. J Clin Endocrinol Metab 2004;89(1):103–7.
44. Buckler JM. Skeletal age changes in puberty. Arch Dis Child 1984;59(2):115–9.
45. Ontell FK, Ivanovic M, Ablin DS, et al. Bone age in children of diverse ethnicity. AJR Am J Roentgenol 1996;167(6):1395–8.
46. Marshall WA. Interrelationships of skeletal maturation, sexual development and somatic growth in man. Ann Hum Biol 1974;1(1):29–40.
47. Flor-Cisneros A, Roemmich JN, Rogol AD, et al. Bone age and onset of puberty in normal boys. Mol Cell Endocrinol 2006;25:254–55;202–6.
48. Klein KO, Larmore KA, de Lancey E, et al. Effect of obesity on estradiol level, and its relationship to leptin, bone maturation, and bone mineral density in children. J Clin Endocrinol Metab 1998;83(10):3469–75.
49. Lazar L, Lebenthal Y, Shalitin S, et al. Natural history of idiopathic advanced bone age diagnosed in childhood: pattern of growth and puberty. Horm Res Paediatr 2011;75(1):49–55.
50. de Waal WJ, Greyn-Fokker MH, Stijnen T, et al. Accuracy of final height prediction and effect of growth-reductive therapy in 362 constitutionally tall children. J Clin Endocrinol Metab 1996;81(3):1206–16.

51. Carel JC, Hay F, Coutant R, et al. Gonadotropin-releasing hormone agonist treatment of girls with constitutional short stature and normal pubertal development. J Clin Endocrinol Metab 1996;81(9):3318–22.
52. Yanovski JA, Rose SR, Municchi G, et al. Treatment with a luteinizing hormone-releasing hormone agonist in adolescents with short stature. N Engl J Med 2003;348(10):908–17.
53. Lanes R, Gunczler P. Final height after combined growth hormone and gonadotrophin-releasing hormone analogue therapy in short healthy children entering into normally timed puberty. Clin Endocrinol (Oxf) 1998;49(2):197–202.
54. Pasquino AM, Pucarelli I, Roggini M, et al. Adult height in short normal girls treated with gonadotropin-releasing hormone analogs and growth hormone. J Clin Endocrinol Metab 2000;85(2):619–22.
55. van Gool SA, Kamp GA, Visser-van Balen H, et al. Final height outcome after three years of growth hormone and gonadotropin-releasing hormone agonist treatment in short adolescents with relatively early puberty. J Clin Endocrinol Metab 2007;92(4):1402–8.
56. Hero M, Norjavaara E, Dunkel L. Inhibition of estrogen biosynthesis with a potent aromatase inhibitor increases predicted adult height in boys with idiopathic short stature: a randomized controlled trial. J Clin Endocrinol Metab 2005;90(12): 6396–402.
57. Hero M, Toiviainen-Salo S, Wickman S, et al. Vertebral morphology in aromatase inhibitor-treated males with idiopathic short stature or constitutional delay of puberty. J Bone Miner Res 2010;25(7):1536–43.
58. Drop SL, De Waal WJ, De Muinck Keizer-Schrama SM. Sex steroid treatment of constitutionally tall stature. Endocr Rev 1998;19(5):540–58.
59. Fontoura M, Brauner R, Prevot C, et al. Precocious puberty in girls: early diagnosis of a slowly progressing variant. Arch Dis Child 1989;64(8):1170–6.
60. Palmert MR, Malin HV, Boepple PA. Unsustained or slowly progressive puberty in young girls: initial presentation and long-term follow-up of 20 untreated patients. J Clin Endocrinol Metab 1999;84(2):415–23.
61. Klein KO. Precocious puberty: who has it? Who should be treated? J Clin Endocrinol Metab 1999;84(2):411–4.
62. Lazar L, Pertzelan A, Weintrob N, et al. Sexual precocity in boys: accelerated versus slowly progressive puberty gonadotropin-suppressive therapy and final height. J Clin Endocrinol Metab 2001;86(9):4127–32.
63. Kauli R, Galatzer A, Kornreich L, et al. Final height of girls with central precocious puberty, untreated versus treated with cyproterone acetate or GnRH analogue. A comparative study with re-evaluation of predictions by the Bayley-Pinneau method. Horm Res 1997;47(2):54–61.
64. Brito VN, Latronico AC, Cukier P, et al. Factors determining normal adult height in girls with gonadotropin-dependent precocious puberty treated with depot gonadotropin-releasing hormone analogs. J Clin Endocrinol Metab 2008;93(7): 2662–9.
65. Bar A, Linder B, Sobel EH, et al. Bayley-Pinneau method of height prediction in girls with central precocious puberty: correlation with adult height. J Pediatr 1995;126(6):955–8.
66. Leger J, Reynaud R, Czernichow P. Do all girls with apparent idiopathic precocious puberty require gonadotropin-releasing hormone agonist treatment? J Pediatr 2000;137(6):819–25.
67. Paul DL, Conte FA, Grumbach MM, et al. Long term effect of gonadotropin-releasing hormone agonist therapy in children with true precocious puberty

treated at a median age of less than 5 years. J Clin Endocrinol Metab 1995;80(2): 546–51.

68. Kletter GB, Kelch RP. Clinical review 60. Effects of gonadotropin-releasing hormone analog therapy on adult stature in precocious puberty. J Clin Endocrinol Metab 1994;79(2):331–4.

69. Arrigo T, Cisternino M, Galluzzi F, et al. Analysis of the factors affecting auxological response to GnRH agonist treatment and final height outcome in girls with idiopathic central precocious puberty. Eur J Endocrinol 1999;141(2):140–4.

70. Oostdijk W, Rikken B, Schreuder S, et al. Final height in central precocious puberty after long term treatment with a slow release GnRH agonist. Arch Dis Child 1996;75(4):292–7.

71. Galluzzi F, Salti R, Bindi G, et al. Adult height comparison between boys and girls with precocious puberty after long-term gonadotrophin-releasing hormone analogue therapy. Acta Paediatr 1998;87(5):521–7.

72. Carel JC, Roger M, Ispas S, et al. French study group of Decapeptyl in precocious puberty Final height after long-term treatment with triptorelin slow release for central precocious puberty: importance of statural growth after interruption of treatment. J Clin Endocrinol Metab 1999;84(6):1973–8.

73. Klein KO, Barnes KM, Jones JV, et al. Increased final height in precocious puberty after long-term treatment with LHRH agonists: the National Institutes of Health experience. J Clin Endocrinol Metab 2001;86(10):4711–6.

74. Lazar L, Padoa A, Phillip M. Growth pattern and final height after cessation of gonadotropin-suppressive therapy in girls with central sexual precocity. J Clin Endocrinol Metab 2007;92(9):3483–9.

75. Cassio A, Cacciari E, Balsamo A, et al. Randomized trial of LHRH analogue treatment on final height in girls with onset of puberty aged 7.5-8.5 years. Arch Dis Child 1999;81(4):329–32.

76. Bouvattier C, Coste J, Rodrigue D, et al. Lack of effect of GnRH agonists on final height in girls with advanced puberty: a randomized long-term pilot study. J Clin Endocrinol Metab 1999;84(1):3575–8.

77. Lazar L, Kauli R, Pertzelan A, et al. Gonadotropin-suppressive therapy in girls with early and fast puberty affects the pace of puberty but not total pubertal growth or final height. J Clin Endocrinol Metab 2002;87(5):2090–4.

78. Mul D, Bertelloni S, Carel JC, et al. Effect of gonadotropin-releasing hormone agonist treatment in boys with central precocious puberty: final height results. Horm Res 2002;58(1):1–7.

79. de Vries L, Guz-Mark A, Lazar L, et al. Premature thelarche: age at presentation affects clinical course but not clinical characteristics or risk to progress to precocious puberty. J Pediatr 2010;156(3):466–71.

80. Oron T, Lebenthal Y, de Vries L, et al. Interrelationship of extent of precocious adrenarche in appropriate for gestational age girls with clinical outcome. J Pediatr 2012;160(2):308–13.

81. Rosenfield RL. Clinical review 6: diagnosis and management of delayed puberty. J Clin Endocrinol Metab 1990;70(3):559–62.

82. Davenport ML. Approach to the patient with Turner syndrome. J clin Endocrinol Metab 2010;95(4):1487–95.

83. Crowne EC, Shalet SM, Wallace WH, et al. Final height in boys with untreated constitutional delay in growth and puberty. Arch Dis Child 1990;65(10):1109–12.

84. Albanese A, Stanhope R. Predictive factors in the determination of final height in boys with constitutional delay of growth and puberty. J Pediatr 1995;126(4): 545–50.

85. Strickland AL, Underwood LE, Voina SJ, et al. Growth retardation in Cushing's syndrome. Am J Dis Child 1972;123(3):207–13.
86. Lee JM, Kaciroti N, Appugliese D, et al. Body mass index and timing of pubertal initiation in boys. Arch Pediatr Adolesc Med 2010;164(2):139–44.
87. Savage MO, Preece MA, Cameron N, et al. Gonadotrophin response to LH-RH in boys with delayed growth and adolescence. Arch Dis Child 1981;56(7):552–6.
88. Zachmann M, Studer S, Prader A. Short-term testosterone treatment at bone age of 12 to 13 years does not reduce adult height in boys with constitutional delay of growth and adolescence. Helv Paediatr Acta 1987;42(1):21–8.
89. Wilson DM, Kei J, Hintz RL, et al. Effects of testosterone therapy for pubertal delay. Am J Dis Child 1988;142(1):96–9.
90. Kelly BP, Paterson WF, Donaldson MD. Final height outcome and value of height prediction in boys with constitutional delay in growth and adolescence treated with intramuscular testosterone 125 mg per month for 3 months. Clin Endocrinol (Oxf) 2003;58(3):267–72.
91. Wehkalampi K, Päkkilä K, Laine T, et al. Adult height in girls with delayed pubertal growth. Horm Res Paediatr 2011;76(2):130–5.
92. Krajewska-Siuda E, Malecka-Tendera E, Krajewski-Siuda K. Are short boys with constitutional delay of growth and puberty candidates for rGH therapy according to FDA recommendations? Horm Res 2006;65(4):192–6.
93. Hero M, Wickman S, Dunkel L. Treatment with the aromatase inhibitor letrozole during adolescence increases near-final height in boys with constitutional delay of puberty. Clin Endocrinol (Oxf) 2006;64(5):510–3.
94. Shulman DI, Francis GL, Palmert MR, et al. Use of aromatase inhibitors in children and adolescents with disorders of growth and adolescent development. Pediatr 2008;121(4):e975–83.
95. Quigley CA, Crowe BJ, Anglin DG, et al. Growth hormone and low dose estrogen in Turner syndrome: results of a United States multi-center trial to near-final height. J Clin Endocrinol Metab 2002;87(5):2033–41.
96. Sperlich M, Butenandt O, Schwarz HP. Final height and predicted height in boys with untreated constitutional growth delay. Eur J Pediatr 1995;154(8):627–32.

Index

Note: Page numbers of article titles are in **boldface** type.

A

Accelerator hypothesis, of type 1 diabetes risk, in children, 690
ACTH. See *Adrenocorticotropin hormone (ACTH)*.
Actions, ADHD effect on, 765–766
Activation, of brain, ADHD effect on, 765–766
ADHD. See *Attention-deficit/hyperactivity disorder (ADHD)*.
Adrenal enzyme inhibitors, for Cushing syndrome, 800–801
Adrenal hyperplasia, massive macronodular, Cushing syndrome associated with, 795
Adrenal tumors, Cushing syndrome related to, 795
    diagnostic techniques for, 797, 799
    treatment of, 800–801
Adrenalectomy, for Cushing syndrome, bilateral total, 800–801
    unilateral, glucocorticoid replacement following, 801
Adrenarche, precocious, 816–817
Adrenergic dysregulation theory, of ADHD, 767–768
Adrenergic neurons, GHRH secretion role, 768–769
Adrenocorticotropin hormone (ACTH), HPA axis regulation of, 793
  in Cushing syndrome, diagnostic tests for, 796–799
    etiology of, 794
Adrenocorticotropin hormone plasma level, in Cushing syndrome diagnosis, single midnight
  measurement of, 797–799
    spot morning measurement of, 798
Adult height, compromised, 713–714, 727
    syndromes of. See *Noonan syndrome (NS); Turner syndrome (TS)*.
    therapy for. See *Human growth hormone (hGH) therapy*.
Adult height prediction (AHP), pubertal disorders and, 806
    BA as functional marker for, 808–809
    normal puberty vs., 812
Adult survivors of cancer, safety of growth hormone therapy in, 789–790
Adverse events, of growth hormone therapy, in children with chronic diseases, 753–754
Age at onset, of type 1 diabetes in children, incidence rates based on, 682, 684
AIP gene, in Cushing syndrome, 795
AIRE-1 gene, in Down syndrome, autoimmune hypothyroidism related to, 741
Alloimmune response, to β-cell replacement, 704
Amino acids, as neurotransmitters, 767
Aminoglutethimide, for Cushing syndrome, 801
Anabolic steroids, for Turner syndrome, 720, 722
Anakinra, for type 1 diabetes, 702
Androgen, bone growth regulation role, during puberty, 809–810
Animal models, for T1D clinical testing, 697, 707–708
Anti-CD3, as type 1 diabetes intervention, 699–700
Anti-CD20, as type 1 diabetes intervention, 700

Endocrinol Metab Clin N Am 41 (2012) 827–850
http://dx.doi.org/10.1016/S0889-8529(12)00115-6
0889-8529/12/$ – see front matter © 2012 Elsevier Inc. All rights reserved.

endo.theclinics.com

1. Publication Title	2. Publication Number	3. Filing Date
Endocrinology and Metabolism Clinics of North America	0 0 0 - 2 7 7 5	9/14/12

4. Issue Frequency	5. Number of Issues Published Annually	6. Annual Subscription Price
Mar, Jun, Sep, Dec	4	$313.00

7. Complete Mailing Address of Known Office of Publication (*Not printer*) (*Street, city, county, state, and ZIP+4®*)

Elsevier Inc.
360 Park Avenue South
New York, NY 10010-1710

Contact Person
Stephen R. Bushing

Telephone (Include area code)
215-239-3688

8. Complete Mailing Address of Headquarters or General Business Office of Publisher (*Not printer*)

Elsevier Inc., 360 Park Avenue South, New York, NY 10010-1710

9. Full Names and Complete Mailing Addresses of Publisher, Editor, and Managing Editor (*Do not leave blank*)

Publisher (*Name and complete mailing address*)

Kim Murphy, Elsevier, Inc., 1600 John F. Kennedy Blvd. Suite 1800, Philadelphia, PA 19103-2899

Editor (*Name and complete mailing address*)

Pamela Hetherington, Elsevier, Inc., 1600 John F. Kennedy Blvd. Suite 1800, Philadelphia, PA 19103-2899

Managing Editor (*Name and complete mailing address*)

Sarah Barth, Elsevier, Inc., 1600 John F. Kennedy Blvd. Suite 1800, Philadelphia, PA 19103-2899

10. Owner (*Do not leave blank. If the publication is owned by a corporation, give the name and address of the corporation immediately followed by the names and addresses of all stockholders owning or holding 1 percent or more of the total amount of stock. If not owned by a corporation, give the names and addresses of the individual owners. If owned by a partnership or other unincorporated firm, give its name and address as well as those of each individual owner. If the publication is published by a nonprofit organization, give its name and address.*)

Full Name	Complete Mailing Address
Wholly owned subsidiary of	1600 John F. Kennedy Blvd., Ste. 1800
Reed/Elsevier, US holdings	Philadelphia, PA 19103-2899

11. Known Bondholders, Mortgagees, and Other Security Holders Owning or Holding 1 Percent or More of Total Amount of Bonds, Mortgages, or Other Securities. If none, check box ☐ None

Full Name	Complete Mailing Address
N/A	

12. Tax Status (*For completion by nonprofit organizations authorized to mail at nonprofit rates*) (*Check one*)
The purpose, function, and nonprofit status of this organization and the exempt status for federal income tax purposes:
☐ Has Not Changed During Preceding 12 Months
☐ Has Changed During Preceding 12 Months (*Publisher must submit explanation of change with this statement*)

PS Form 3526, September 2007 (Page 1 of 3 (Instructions Page 3)) PSN 7530-01-000-9931 **PRIVACY NOTICE**: See our Privacy policy in www.usps.com

13. Publication Title	14. Issue Date for Circulation Data Below
Endocrinology and Metabolism Clinics of North America	September 2012

15. Extent and Nature of Circulation			Average No. Copies Each Issue During Preceding 12 Months	No. Copies of Single Issue Published Nearest to Filing Date
a. Total Number of Copies (*Net press run*)			1292	1060
b. Paid Circulation (By Mail and Outside the Mail)	(1)	Mailed Outside-County Paid Subscriptions Stated on PS Form 3541 (*Include paid distribution above nominal rate, advertiser's proof copies, and exchange copies*)	483	435
	(2)	Mailed In-County Paid Subscriptions Stated on PS Form 3541 (*Include paid distribution above nominal rate, advertiser's proof copies, and exchange copies*)		
	(3)	Paid Distribution Outside the Mails Including Sales Through Dealers and Carriers, Street Vendors, Counter Sales, and Other Paid Distribution Outside USPS®	375	351
	(4)	Paid Distribution by Other Classes Mailed Through the USPS (e.g. First-Class Mail®)		
c. Total Paid Distribution (Sum of 15b (1), (2), (3), and (4))			858	786
d. Free or Nominal Rate Distribution (By Mail and Outside the Mail)	(1)	Free or Nominal Rate Outside-County Copies Included on PS Form 3541	75	71
	(2)	Free or Nominal Rate In-County Copies Included on PS Form 3541		
	(3)	Free or Nominal Rate Copies Mailed at Other Classes Through the USPS (e.g. First-Class Mail)		
	(4)	Free or Nominal Rate Distribution Outside the Mail (Carriers or other means)		
e. Total Free or Nominal Rate Distribution (Sum of 15d (1), (2), (3) and (4))			75	71
f. Total Distribution (Sum of 15c and 15e)			933	857
g. Copies not Distributed (See instructions to publishers #4 (page #3))			359	203
h. Total (Sum of 15f and g)			1292	1060
i. Percent Paid (15c divided by 15f times 100)			91.96%	91.72%

16. Publication of Statement of Ownership

If the publication is a general publication, publication of this statement is required. Will be printed ☐ Publication not required
in the **December 2012** issue of this publication.

17. Signature and Title of Editor, Publisher, Business Manager, or Owner

Stephen R. Bushing Inventory Distribution Coordinator Date September 14, 2012

I certify that all information furnished on this form is true and complete. I understand that anyone who furnishes false or misleading information on this form or who omits material or information requested on the form may be subject to criminal sanctions (including fines and imprisonment) and/or civil sanctions (including civil penalties)

PS Form 3526, September 2007 (Page 2 of 3)